Men'sHealth

BEST.
SEX.
EVER.

Men'sHealth

BEST.
SEX.
EVER.

200 Frank, Funny & Friendly Answers About **Getting It On**

With **65 life-changing positions** illustrated in *great* detail

Jordyn Taylor & Zachary Zane

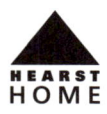

HEARST HOME

CONTENTS

foreword by Justin Lehmiller
6

introduction
8

meet your authors
11

index
197

BEST. SEX. EVER.

CHAPTER 1
Warming Up
13

CHAPTER 2
Talk Dirty to Me
31

CHAPTER 3
Doin' It
47

CHAPTER 4
What's Up With My Junk?
73

CHAPTER 5
Butt Stuff
95

CHAPTER 6
Kinks and Fetishes
119

CHAPTER 7
Self-Love
145

CHAPTER 8
The Climax
165

CHAPTER 9
Closing Lines
181

FOREWORD

Why Do Human Beings Have Sex?

Scientists have uncovered at least 237 distinct reasons, but there's one that tops the list across gender, sexual orientation, and age: *pleasure*. That's right—the single biggest thing that leads us to pursue sex is that it feels good.

As someone who has spent most of their adult life as a sex educator, I therefore find it strange (and disappointing) that most of the education people receive around sex neglects pleasure entirely. Far too many of us never heard a peep about pleasure when we learned about sex and, instead, were taught that sex serves just one purpose—procreation.

However, procreation is actually one of the *least* common reasons people have sex. Likewise, there are plenty of sexually active people who will never once engage in procreative sex. We need sex ed that doesn't disconnect sex from its core motivation.

That's why I'm thrilled to be part of *Best. Sex. Ever.* It's the sex ed you always needed but never received—and it can help you unlock the pleasure you've been seeking.

While this book runs the gamut of topics, including everything from kissing and oral sex to dirty talk and kink, a few broad themes run throughout. They represent a tried and true "recipe" for leveling up your sex life and keeping passion alive in long-term relationships. The three key ingredients are as follows:

BEST. SEX. EVER.

1. *Good sex is all about good communication.* As I say in my own book *Tell Me What You Want*, "people find it more challenging to talk about sex than to actually have it." When we can't communicate effectively about sex, it creates a massive barrier to pleasure because it puts your partner in the position of having to read your mind and guess what you do and don't like in the bedroom. In the pages ahead, you'll learn how to start healthy sexual conversations and confidently express your fantasies and desires.

2. *You can't tell your partner what you want if you don't know what you like.* Everyone's body works a little differently. For example, some people can orgasm just from having their nipples played with, while others get next to nothing out of this. Masturbation and self-exploration can help you understand what works best for you. This book will help you document your own road map to pleasure, including the shortcuts and long-haul trips, so that you can effectively guide your partner to your preferred sexual destination.

3. *Variety is the spice of your sex life.* One of the most consistent findings in sex research is that the most sexually satisfied people have the most expansive definitions of sex and are constantly trying new things. This makes sense because novelty makes it easier to get—and stay—in the mood, while also intensifying pleasure. Whether you're new to sex or think you've tried it all, you'll find plenty of inspiration ahead.

Commit these to memory and enjoy the best sex *ever*!

Justin Lehmiller
Men's Health advisory panel member, a research fellow at the Kinsey Institute, and the author of *Tell Me What You Want*

INTRODUCTION

We made a bold promise with the title of this book.

The best sex...ever? What does that even mean?

Take a few seconds to pause and picture your dream sexual scenario. Maybe it's silk sheets and rose petals and chocolate-dipped strawberries. Maybe it's handcuffs and a blindfold and "Who's your daddy?" Maybe it's a threesome or a foursome or, hell, a full-blown ancient-Rome-bacchanal-style orgy. Or maybe it's sexy solo time with some porn and your favorite booty toy. By all means, let your fantasies run wild. As long as it's safe and consensual, we here at *Men's Health* do not judge.

We all have different bodies, orientations, comfort levels, and kinks in the bedroom (or wherever you like to get it on), which is why the last thing we want to do is tell you what kind of sex you should be having. What we're trying to say is, there's no one scenario that makes for the best sex ever. *Whatever* sex you have when you feel free and empowered to explore your deepest desires is the Best. Sex. Ever.

But if that were easy to achieve, we wouldn't have had to write a whole book on it. Unfortunately, many of us grew up with—and still carry the weight

INTRODUCTION

of—sexual shame and insufficient sex education. (FYI, as of September 1, 2021, only 15 states are required to teach sex education that is medically accurate.) And even where sex ed is taught, it tends to be hella heteronormative.

From the moment an adult first lies to us about where babies come from, we begin to internalize sex negativity, i.e., the false belief that sex is inherently dirty and wrong. We're bombarded with sex-negative messages from, well, everywhere. Some of us grew up in a religion that told us sex is *only* between a cisgender man and woman and for the sole purpose of procreation. Some of our parents told us that masturbating every day made us perverts. And some of us had a health teacher who scared the crap out of us with a lecture on sexually transmitted infections. Even if you didn't have one defining shameful experience, it's hard to escape the sex negativity that still runs rampant in our society, from political legislation to reality TV dating shows.

Bombarded by all this negative and downright inaccurate messaging, many of us are left afraid to embrace our sexual identity and desires—or even

BEST. SEX. EVER.

talk about sex, for that matter. Not only are we left feeling embarrassed by our sexual desires, but we also don't even know what's healthy or normal.

Well, that's where we come in.

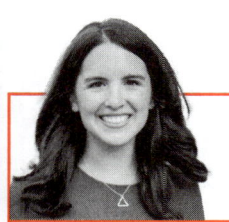

MEET YOUR AUTHORS

Jordyn Taylor

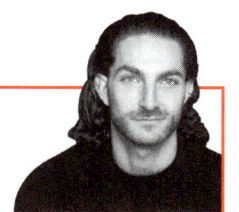

I'm the deputy digital editor at *Men's Health*, where the biggest (and best!) part of my job is directing the sex and relationships coverage you see on our website and in our magazine. My goal, through the stories we publish, is to help guys enjoy their sex and love lives without shame holding them back.

I've worked as a reporter and editor covering health, sex, relationships, and LGBTQ+ issues since 2012. I've interviewed countless experts from condom scientists to porn performers, received a journalism fellowship to report on HIV/AIDS, and tested approximately one billion sex toys, which are currently bursting out of every available drawer in my New York City apartment.

My work has also been published by the *New York Observer*, *Mic*, and Glamour.com, and I'm an adjunct professor of journalism at New York University's Arthur L. Carter Journalism Institute.

Zachary Zane

According to the *NY Daily News*, I'm a "bisexual mega-influencer," but I describe myself as a sex-positive, polyamorous kinkster. I also write the *Men's Health* weekly sex advice column, "Sexplain It."

I have a quarterly column at *Queer Majority* titled "Zach and the City," which explores romance and sexuality through my adventurous life. It's set against the backdrop of New York City, and I use my personal experiences as a daring socialite to unpack the current state of cosmopolitan sex, love, and dating.

I've written about sex for the *New York Times*, *Rolling Stone*, the *Washington Post*, *Cosmo*, the *Daily Beast*, NBC, *GQ*, *Allure*, *Slate*, *Playboy*, *Bustle*, *Prevention*, and *AskMen*, among others.

While not writing, speaking, or thinking about sex, I'm likely gettin' some—usually in a New York Sports Club sauna with a married "straight" man.

INTRODUCTION

With the wisdom of the sex experts who advised us on each chapter—you'll meet them as you read through the book—we're going to help you reach a point where you're not ashamed to embrace your sexual desires. We're also going to give you medically accurate tips and techniques for maximizing your pleasure (hi, multiple orgasms) and dive deep into questions you've been too afraid to ask, like: Is dirty talk problematic in a #MeToo world? Is it weird that a straight dude kinda wants to try prostate massage? And WTF is jelqing?

This isn't the toxic sex talk you've heard in the gym locker room or the terrifying lecture you got in high school sex ed. This is the open-minded, sex-positive, and shame-free guide to turning whatever fantasy you pictured a few minutes ago into a reality.

Welcome to the first day of the rest of your sex life.

BEST. SEX. EVER.

YOUR SEXPERT

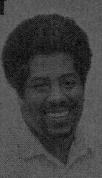

Jor-El Caraballo is a licensed mental health counselor and an educator who presents on consent and healthy sexuality.

1

WARMING UP

Let's start at the very beginning, from asking for consent (at every stage of a hookup!) to initiating sex when it's *checks calendar* been a while.

CHAPTER

WARMING UP

Where's the Line Between Flirty and Creepy?

Do you have tips for a well-meaning guy who wants to approach a sexy stranger without coming off as creepy?
Caraballo: Um, yes and no. No because the reality is, whether they're approaching women or other men, there's almost this default assumption that men are creepy.

Which is justified! How should that underlying dynamic inform guys' behavior in these situations?
Be aware of your presence, knowing you might be perceived in a certain way, and just try and start softly—even something as simple as introducing yourself and inviting a conversation, not mandating one. This is where I'm not too fond of dating coaches. They'll say, "Get in there! Be confident! Take up that space!" And the problem with that is it's already starting this dynamic in which one person is dictating consent.

But what if you approached the situation and said, "Hey, I saw you sitting there and thought you looked interesting. Would you like to chat? My name is so-and-so"? You're creating this dynamic in which this person feels safer because you're introducing the concepts of consent and agency in a way you wouldn't be otherwise.

Telling someone you're interested can be nerve-racking. How can guys project more confidence going into a sexual scenario?
You can't project confidence if you don't have it. We have to move away from that being an "act" to something we recognize is really an inside job. This whole "fake it till you make it" saying might be okay for a moment—you might be able to white-knuckle that—but it's important to really do the inner work, to figure out "What's keeping me from feeling confident, and how do I work through that?" instead of just trying to "project" confidence in order to get some prize of another person.

Great point. Rephrasing the question: What can men do to feel more confident from within?
Ongoing self-reflection. It can look like therapy or self-help books or digital courses on managing stress and anxiety. Start to do the work. And as you continue to work through it and you start to see success, you'll start to feel more confident—because that's another thing you've accomplished that's really important! You've worked on yourself and bettered yourself as a whole person, and that will make you a better partner.

WARMING UP

What's Enthusiastic Consent?

Hey there. We noticed you reading this book and thought you looked interesting. We'd love to tell you all about kicking off a sexy encounter. How would you feel about that?

All sexual activity (touching, kissing, intercourse, you name it) must begin with explicit eagerness from everyone taking part. Not only is it *the law*, but trust us, hooking up is way more fun when all parties are equally into it too.

Imagine you're inviting a friend out to dinner next Friday, Caraballo says. How would you feel if their response were "I guess so…that's all right" versus "Oh, yeah! We can go to this place I heard about!" "That already makes the experience much more enjoyable and richer," he points out.

Depending on when you last took a sex ed class, you might remember the saying "no means no"—in other words, you have to stop whatever you're doing if your partner objects to it. Which is true! But the problem with "no means no" is it implies that the *lack* of an objection, like a noncommittal shrug or straight-up silence, is a green light to keep going. Seems dicey, right?

The current (and much better!) way of thinking is "yes means yes." It's known as *enthusiastic consent*—you might have heard the term before. If not, think of it as a "fuck yes" to sexual activity, Caraballo says. Anything else is a no. "Enthusiastic consent is having an overtly and explicitly clear indication that the person wants to move forward with whatever's happening, to the point that there is no room for doubt," he says. "It also has to be verbal."

How Do I Ask for Enthusiastic Consent?

There's a common misconception that obtaining consent has to be uncomfortably formal, like you're a lawyer asking your partner to initial a contract here…here…and here. Wrong! "It could be something that's actually very sexy," Caraballo says. "A lot of people respond well to dirty talk in some form, and this can lend itself to that."

That said, if you're not used to asking for consent, it might feel a little awkward the first few times you do it, just like any new thing you try in the bedroom. But the more you do it, the easier it gets. And besides, "it's so much better to suffer through a few moments of awkwardness than the alternative," Caraballo adds. "The alternative is that there's actually been serious harm done."

You don't want that! To help ease the awkwardness, here are some sample questions to get you started. Remember: Whether you're with a new partner or someone you've been with for years, you want to keep the communication flowing throughout the whole session.

- *"Can I kiss your beautiful lips?"*
- *"How far do you want to go tonight?"*
- *"Can I help you undress?"*
- *"Do you want to unbutton this for me?"*
- *"Does this feel good?"*
- *"Do you want me to keep going?"*
- *"I bet you taste so good. Can I go down on you?"*
- *"I'm really into role play. Is that something you'd want to try tonight?"*
- *"Are you okay with me touching that sexy ass of yours?"*
- *"Do you want me to grab a condom?"*
- *"How would you like to feel me inside of you?"*
- *"Do you want to try using this vibrator together?"*
- *"Where do you want me to finish?"*

WARMING UP

Ask what language affirms your partner.

Besides getting consent, you also want to learn: "What would make this hookup the best possible sexual experience for you?" That includes asking about affirming language, says NYC-based psychotherapist and sex therapist Dulcinea Alex Pitagora, Ph.D., LSCW, CST.

"For some trans men who have dysphoria about having a vagina (which some might feel fine calling it a vagina, and some might call it a front hole or use another name, or they may avoid referring to it at all), receiving penetrative sex could be triggering, and remind them of a body part they would rather not have," Pitagora says. "Some trans men who are bottoms might enjoy receptive anal sex but not enjoy receptive vaginal sex for that reason. Again, all of this is on a case-by-case basis, and it's never wise to make assumptions, but to ask conscientiously and in a way that doesn't sound fetishizing."

An example of this would be, "Do you feel like talking about what feels and sounds good to you during sex?" and "Are there words or types of sex that really turn you on, or that you want me to avoid because it really turns you off?"

Pro Tip: ➡ If You're Unsure, Stop!

If they say they're into it but their body language indicates otherwise—maybe they're tense, limp, avoiding eye contact, or pulling away from you—stop what you're doing, move off or away from your partner, and reassess the situation. "Your presence physically, even if you don't intend it to be, can be intimidating," Caraballo says. So if your partner seems tense, go ahead and say, "Hey, you seem a little uncomfortable, let's take a step back." Then stop what you're doing and go back to talking. Keep in mind that alcohol and other mind-altering substances can make it harder to read those subtle cues that something's off.

BEST. SEX. EVER.

What Are the Keys to Good Kissing?

Everyone's heard a story about a make-out gone wrong: a guy who bit his partner's lip so hard they needed stitches or a teenage couple whose braces got stuck together mid-smooch. There's no doubt some of them are urban legends, but the fact remains that knowing how to kiss is a valuable skill. A good make-out sesh can be romantic as hell on its own or a nifty first step in your foreplay routine.

"When we kiss, we release oxytocin, a bonding chemical, which makes us feel closer and prepares us for intimacy," says our Chapter 8 sexpert, sex educator Kenneth Play. "The lips and tongue have tons of nerve endings, and sharing them gives us an incredible, sensorially rich experience."

Here are some tips for kissing like a pro. (That said, remember that everyone kisses differently, and it might take a minute to sync up with your partner!)

Pay attention to your partner's cues.

This applies to all aspects of making out, from the depth of your tongue to what you're doing with your hands. If your partner moans with pleasure, mirrors your moves, or gives another form of positive feedback, it's a good indication that you should keep going. If they pull away or decline to reciprocate your actions, maybe it's time to change tack or stop and check in.

The key is *moving slowly* so you can register their reactions and respond accordingly. Do not—we repeat, *do not*—go in with your mouth wide open (unless you have kissed this person before and know they're into that kind of thing). Start with a soft, tongue-free kiss and gradually move deeper when you're both ready.

Keep your tongue and lips soft.

"No one likes to be jabbed with a pointy tongue," Play says. Practice moving your tongue around without tensing it up and turning it into a rock.

Speaking of jabbing, don't thrust your tongue like a jackhammer! Instead, take a gentler approach. "Wherever it is that you meet with the tongues, a good way of doing things is to think of massaging [their] tongue with yours gently," Play says.

Mix up the depth of your kiss.

Remember to read those cues. If your partner is signaling they'd like your tongue to go deeper—think pulling the back of your neck or head toward them or opening their mouth wider—then feel free to gently roam further. Just make sure you don't *stay* back there.

"It's the mixture between types of kisses and the dance between deep and shallow that usually makes for the best make-outs," Play says. "Like music, you want to dance through a symphony of different notes—high, medium, and low—and different rhythms to make for the best experience."

Try biting or sucking—carefully.

For the love of all things holy, don't chomp down on your partner's lip like you're taking a bite of a sandwich. Start with a little sucking and soft nibbling, and read their cues from there.

Get their hair involved.

"Pulling [their] hair can feel nice if it's done right," Play says. "Grab a big handful and squeeze, rather than pulling [their] head backward. The more hair in your hand, the less likely it is to actually hurt [them]. It will feel like more of a firm pressure against [their] scalp, which displays competence and assertiveness while displaying desire."

Don't forget about eye contact.

"Staring deeply into each other's eyes creates tons of intimacy and lets [them] know you are truly present," Play says. Just make sure you're not locking eyes the whole time, which could potentially come off as creepy.

Can't seem to get in sync with your partner?

It happens. If you just can't find the right rhythm, Play recommends playing a "game" to find out how your partner likes to make out. Tell them to kiss you however they want, and then follow their lead. "This way, you can learn [their] movements," he says. People "will usually kiss you the way [they want] to be kissed."

Pro Tip: ➡ Get Creative With Kissing

Kissing wouldn't be as fun if there were only one way to do it. If you had to peck everyone for the rest of your life, you'd probably be hungry for more passion. But if you could only ever French-kiss, you'd probably get some weird stares out in public. Thankfully, there are *tons* of creative styles out there, including these fun options:

The Ice Kiss Hold an ice chip between your lips when you start making out and try passing it back and forth. Keep kissing until the ice melts!

The Drink Kiss Take a small sip of your beverage and then kiss your partner, transferring the liquid to them. It may seem simple, but it's not—make sure to use only a little bit of liquid, and be prepared to spill.

The Vampire Kiss If your partner's okay with hickeys, move from kissing their lips to gently biting and sucking their neck. It's a super-sensitive erogenous zone!

WARMING UP

CONFESSIONS

"My Funniest First Time Was..."

"My girlfriend and I had a hell of a time figuring out the mechanics of missionary sex. After several frustrating minutes for her, she finally said, 'Forget it,' and flipped me on my back and rode me. At the time, it was embarrassing, but looking back on it almost 30 years later, it makes me giggle." —**Nate, 43**

"I was so nervous, I began to scream and moan before he penetrated me." —**Fernando, 39**

"First time I got a blowjob: As we were taking off our clothes, she tossed in, 'If you leave your socks on, this is all over.' I had no idea people had such strong feelings about socks and sex!" —**David, 29**

"During my first anal experience, I came so hard that I shot cum in my own eye." —**Tom, 50**

"On a first date, we went back to his place. While I was topping [penetrating] him, he said, 'Oh, fuck, I think I love you—I mean, this! I love *this*! Fuck.' We laughed it off, but the sex was great."
—**Gregg, 30**

"My first time having a threesome, the couple was absolutely gorgeous and I felt super comfortable and confident, but my dick was NOT on board. No blood flow at all. I ended up just watching and filming them and loosening up, and we all had a blast anyway. We tried again another time and things went as planned."
—**Matthew, 35**

BEST. SEX. EVER.

We Don't Have Sex as Much as We Used To. How Do We Start Again?

The novelty of a budding romance can make it hard to keep your hands off each other. But as time passes and you settle into your routines, you might notice you're not doin' it like bunnies anymore. "What you're doing is exchanging novelty for comfort and security," Caraballo explains. That said, it's normal to want to have more sex, and the good news is it's never too late to relight that fire, as long as both of you are into it.

"One thing that partners can do is to think about any kind of difference they can inject into their sexual lives together," Caraballo says. "It could be really small, as in a new position or location, or it could be something a bit more adventurous, like a new partner or new toys." (Head to page 68 to see our favorite sex toys for couples!)

How do you tell your partner you want to heat things up again? As with overcoming almost all relationship issues, the key is confronting your bedroom rut as a problem you'll solve together—not pointing fingers and attempting to assign blame. Caraballo suggests that instead of saying: "Hey, our sex life sucks. I don't think you're working hard enough." Try: "Hey, I want to talk to you about something I've been thinking about. What do you think about maybe changing some of the ways we engage sexually?"

"That gives people room to not be as defensive and be more collaborative as you [both] problem-solve and think about things that could happen moving forward," he says.

WARMING UP

Say What Now?

What's the _Honeymoon Phase_?

It's the early stage of a relationship when you prioritize your partner above all else. "Everything just feels lovely and hopeful and exciting and passionate," Caraballo says. "Not to sound cynical, but it's not a completely accurate representation of the relationship." Over time, as you return to balancing work, family, and friends alongside your new romance, you might feel like you're crashing back down to earth—but this doesn't mean your relationship's doomed, Caraballo adds: "It can feel less exciting or passionate but still be the thing that you want."

How Are We Supposed to Have Sex if We're Never in the Mood at the Same Time?

We feel you. Agreeing to get it on would be so much easier if you both got struck by a lightning bolt of horniness at the exact same time. As you've probably figured out by now, there's no way to bribe the lightning gods to make sure you both get turned on simultaneously. However, understanding the patterns of desire that change from person to person, and how to act on them, may help you boost your sexual frequency.

Let's say one of you gets horny every night at 9 p.m., like clockwork, while the other is rarely (if ever) overcome by a sudden urge to bone. You may assume the first person is simply way more interested in sex, but that's not necessarily the case. Instead, it may be that they experience _spontaneous desire_—i.e., horniness that comes out of nowhere—while their partner experiences _responsive desire_—i.e., horniness triggered by some kind of sexy stimulus, like an intimate cuddle sesh or a kiss on the back of the neck. "If those two people just stayed in their corners and operated in the same way they always have, they're probably not going to have a lot of sex," Caraballo says.

When couples have mismatched patterns of desire, Caraballo recommends that the person who's already in the mood approach their partner with the "romantic equivalent of an amuse-bouche" (the name for those delicate little hors d'oeuvres that restaurants sometimes bring you at the start of a meal). "You're helping them awaken that energy, and they might be ready to go after that," he says.

The choice of amuse-bouche should depend on what the "responsive-desire partner" finds sexy. Maybe it's a kiss that lingers a little longer than your usual "welcome home" peck or a hug where your hands do a little extra wandering. Maybe it's sucking on their toes! "It's really about knowing your partner and what they normally would be turned on by and then bringing some version of that as a way to initiate the experience," he says. "Use the past successes, right?"

Pro Tip: ➡ Sometimes the Sex Problem Isn't About Sex

Sometimes a stale sex life stems from issues outside the bedroom. "When people are thinking about being in a sex rut, I ask them to start by reflecting on how the relationship is first: 'How have you been feeling in your connection with this other person?'" Caraballo says. "Sometimes people require a feeling of connection in order to have sex and to engage in that way, and other people use sex to *have* that connection. It's almost ironic that those two people always end up together."

WARMING UP

THE BEST POSITIONS FOR...
WHEN YOU'RE TIRED AF

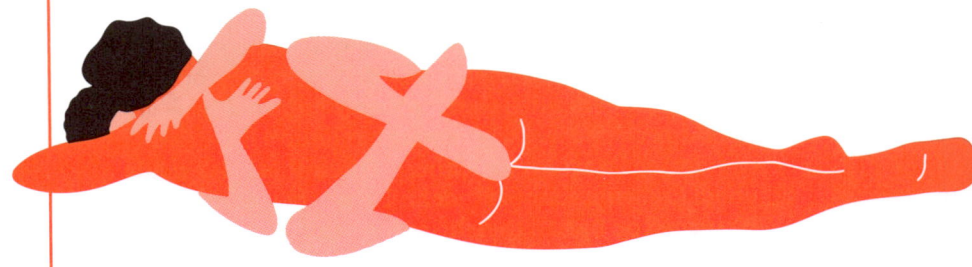

↑ **GIFT WRAPPED**

From missionary, the receiver can wrap their legs around their partner, and then you can both rotate 90 degrees to end up in *this* configuration. Not only is this one relaxing because you're both lying down, but it's also super passionate, with the receiving partner clinging on for dear life.

↑ **LOCKED AND LOADED**

It's like cowgirl...but where the rider gets to lie down, because being on top is tiring! This one's perfect for making out and intimate eye-gazing.

BEST. SEX. EVER.

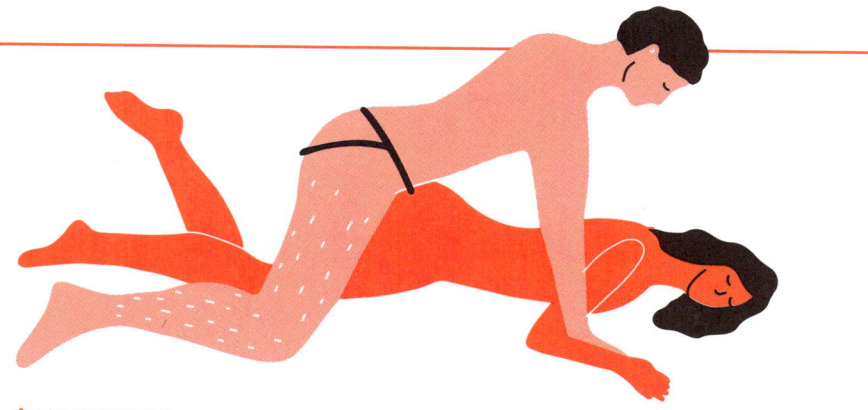

↑ THE FLAT IRON

Especially if you're the receiver, this is as close to a nap as you can get while boning. That said, the delicious sensations of deep penetration will probably keep you both from dozing off.

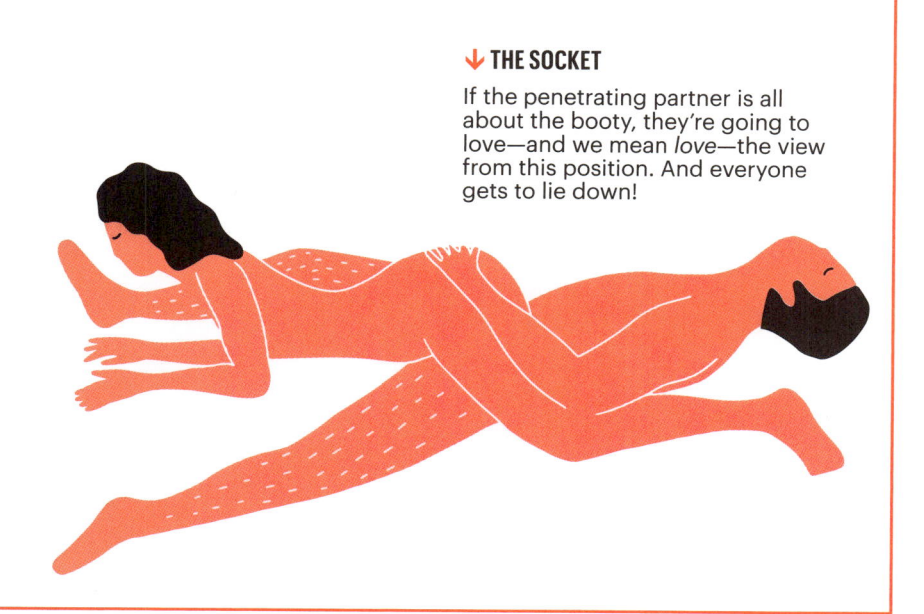

↓ THE SOCKET

If the penetrating partner is all about the booty, they're going to love—and we mean *love*—the view from this position. And everyone gets to lie down!

WARMING UP

SEXPLAIN IT

Dear Sexplain It,

My wife and I had a ton of sex in the first few years we were together, including after we got married. It was almost every day—for years. But a few work promotions and three kids later, everything has changed. My wife and I are swamped with work and family stuff, so we don't have a lot of time for sex (or, frankly, anything romantic at all).

To fix this, my wife wants to add a sex schedule to our shared Google calendar. The idea makes me feel like we've fundamentally failed at something. And I'm not sure I'll enjoy it: I feel like scheduling sex removes all the passion and makes it feel sterile and boring. I guess sex has always been spontaneous for me, so I'm really struggling to wrap my head around making it so...formal. Am I looking at this the wrong way? Is there a way to have passionate sex even when scheduling it?

—Old and Boring

Dear Old and Boring,

You *are* looking at this the wrong way. Here's how I would look at it instead: YOU ARE ABOUT TO HAVE A LOT MORE SEX. Why on earth would you ever complain about that? Actually, let's go ahead and answer that not-so-rhetorical question, because I think it speaks to the root of your discomfort. You clearly have this idea that sex should be spontaneous and passionate. After all, that is how sex is depicted in movies. I'm assuming it's also how things felt toward the beginning of your relationship, which explains why the proposal of a sex schedule feels so jarring to you.

But let's be real: Things change. You're dealing with kids and stressful jobs now. You're older—there's no changing that—but you're not necessarily boring, as your sign-off suggests. Can we stop for a second and appreciate the fact that you both still want to have sex, even with all the obstacles in your life making it more difficult? That's huge! Many couples would just give up. I showed your question to sexuality and relationships scientist Zhana Vrangalova, Ph.D., and I liked how she put it: "You're a prisoner of the unrealistic expectation that sex in long-term relationships needs to happen as spontaneously as it did at the beginning of the relationship."

Right now, it seems like you have this idea that scheduled sex will be stale or unimaginative and that no matter what, it's doomed to be worse than spontaneous sex. Untrue! Scheduled sex can be *better*, because you have time to prepare. "You can plan it, make it special, do different things every time, dress up for each other, seduce each other all over again, start the foreplay the day of by texting and sexting each other, build up the tension, and so on," Vrangalova says. (I'd like to add that this gives you adequate time to charge your sex toys!)

WARMING UP

A personal aside: I want to say that as a bisexual man who has a lot of anal sex, I'm always scheduling sex. Gay men, in general, have to schedule (or at least prepare for) sex because they need to douche and clean their booty prior to the act. Right now, my boyfriend and I are on this threesome spree. These men don't magically fall into our bedroom. (I wish!) We have to schedule a time when all three of us can meet. And the sex has been fucking fabulous because there's another hot dude there who wouldn't be there *unless we scheduled*.

One potential challenge during scheduled sex is getting into the groove. That's because you're not having sex when you're spontaneously horny; rather, you're doing it because you know that sex is good for you, and you like having sex. This brings us back to the responsive desire we talked about earlier in the chapter. "It's basically the desire for sex that we start to feel only after we've started engaging in something sexual that gets our body aroused before the desire in our brain catches on," Vrangalova says. In other words, it may take a few moments for your horniness to set in, and that's totally okay. Just because you're not all hot and bothered the second you touch each other doesn't mean you won't become horned up after a few minutes.

Old and Boring, I'm excited for you. You're about to have a lot more sex, and I bet you're going to enjoy it. Because I can't stop the passage of time, you'll still be Old, but at least you'll be Old and Exciting. Not too shabby!

BEST. SEX. EVER.

YOUR SEXPERT

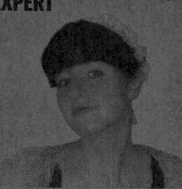

Gigi Engle is a certified sex educator and the author of *All the F*cking Mistakes*.

TALK DIRTY TO ME

2

Learn to make your partner melt with your words alone—and, okay, maybe a few tasteful nudes too.

CHAPTER

TALK DIRTY TO ME

Is Dirty Talk Still Okay in a #MeToo Era?

We know dirty talk is great in theory, but for a lot of guys, it can be scary to put into practice. Why is that?
ENGLE: More than anything, it's fear of rejection. It's kind of scary to wade into waters like that if you're not sure how it's going to be received by a partner. There's a fear of saying the wrong thing or saying something that's too much or not saying the thing your partner wants to hear or being told you're not good at it.

What do you say to clients who come to you with those fears?
First of all, you have to have a conversation with potential partners to acknowledge the fact that you're nervous. There's, like, a 0.005 percent chance that your partner doesn't also feel that way. I mean, I still get embarrassed or nervous when I'm going to talk dirty, and I'm an expert at it. Then it's about communicating with your partner and figuring out what their fantasies and desires are.

Some well-meaning modern men also worry about saying something misogynistic. What's the verdict on using degrading words like *bitch, slut,* and *whore*?
Words like these can be super erotically charged if that's something you're into, and they can also be very threatening and very off-putting depending on the context and the person who's hearing them. You need to know what you're allowed to work with before you just dive headfirst and call someone your "dirty little cock whore." Have the difficult conversations—because you know what's a more difficult conversation than asking

someone if using the word *slut* is okay? Using [it] and finding out later that it wasn't okay.

Should I ask something like, "Is it appropriate if I call you a slut?"
You don't have to say it like that! You can say, "Is there a word that really turns you on? For me, I like it when you talk about my big cock," or "I like it when people call me *daddy* or *sir*." Invite them to tell you their fantasies by offering a couple of yours.

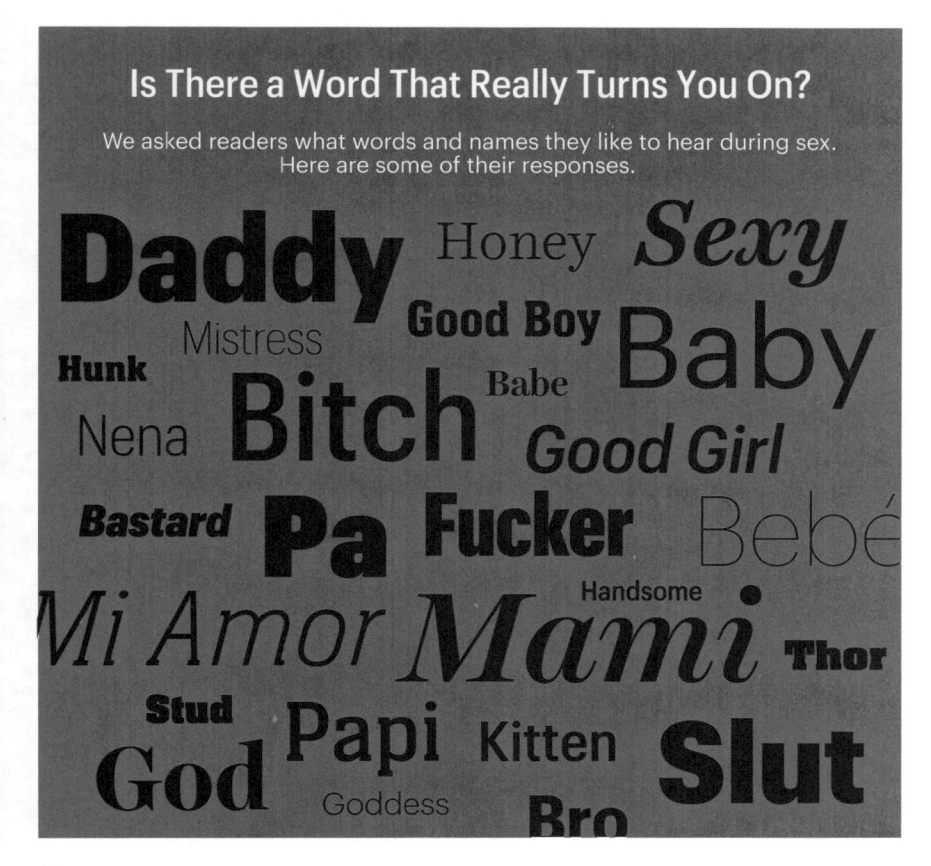

Is There a Word That Really Turns You On?

We asked readers what words and names they like to hear during sex. Here are some of their responses.

Daddy · Honey · Sexy · Mistress · Good Boy · Baby · Hunk · Babe · Nena · Bitch · Good Girl · Bastard · Pa · Fucker · Bebé · Mi Amor · Handsome · Mami · Thor · Stud · God · Papi · Kitten · Slut · Goddess · Bro

TALK DIRTY TO ME

Can I Start With Sexting?

Yes! In fact, if you're dealing with dirty talk stage fright, we recommend it. It's like a dress rehearsal—low pressure—where you get to perform without the audience staring straight back at you. (Plus, if you try something new and they're not into it, it'll feel better getting their feedback via text than when you're standing in their bedroom naked and exposed.)

Even if you're a seasoned pro when it comes to dirty talk, there's so much to love about sexting. Nothing spices up a dull workday like checking your phone and finding out your partner can't wait to bend you over and go to town tonight—and no, it's not just the welcome distraction from Todd's two-hour PowerPoint presentation. Whether you're single and on the apps, casually dating, or in a committed long-term relationship, swapping sexy messages helps build anticipation and fire up your sex drive. If you and a partner spend the day describing exactly what you want to do to each other later, well, just *try* not to rip each other's clothes off the minute you're finally together.

Remember, as with any sexy activity, sexting requires enthusiastic consent (see page 16 if you need a definition). It doesn't have to be formal; you can keep things casual with a message like: "Are you into sexting?" And if they say yes: "Are you down to try it?" If you get the green light, great! But...now what? Do *not* start with a close-up of your junk. Instead, follow these tips for sexting success.

Go easy on the gas.

If you kick things off with a dick pic, there's no room to build. (Also, there are much sexier ways to take naked selfies—see page 40.) Get rolling with something simple, such as describing what you're wearing or what you're "doing" right now.

Try these prompts from Engle:

- "I'm in a suit and tie. I look very put-together. For now."
- "I'm taking off my belt and thinking about you."
- "I'm in that shirt you really like. The blue one."
- "I'm lying in bed naked."
- "I'm touching myself."
- "I'm so turned on right now, thinking about you."

Sext about what you want to do the next time you're together.

"Explaining exactly what you want to do to your partner, whether it's inspired by erotica, porn, or a real-life past sexual experience, is a simplified way to ease into dirty talk without feeling awkward," Engle says.

Try these prompts:

- "I want to strip you naked as soon as I see you."
- "I want to bend you over my desk when you get here."
- "I want to throw you on the bed and have my way with you."

You could even show them the sex toys and props you can't wait to use together. Send a picture of a silky blindfold and tell them you can't wait to tease them until they're begging for more.

TALK DIRTY TO ME

Write a sexy story.

If you fancy yourself a wordsmith or you just have some free time, Engle suggests writing a sexy story (think a paragraph or two—not a novel!) and emailing it to your partner. "Sometimes having a fuller narrative can keep the sexting flow going," she says.

Not sure what to write? Try describing a short fantasy you've always had. Or make it collaborative: Set up a sexy situation and invite them to write the next scene.

Try these prompts:

- *"We're at a nude spa, and we're both getting so turned on from the people around us. We go into a dark, steamy sauna, and there's another attractive couple inside. What happens next?"*
- *"We're in a cabin in the mountains, and it's snowing so hard that we can't go outside. We light a fire in the fireplace. We lie down on the couch. What should we do next?"*
- *"We're strangers who get seated next to each other on a plane. I notice how hot you are, and I can't stop stealing glances at you out of the corner of my eye. You catch me looking at you. What do you do?"*
- *"You and I are hooking up at a sex party, and the hottest person in the room comes over to us and asks to join. What happens from there?"*
- *"We're coworkers who've been into each other for the longest time, and we both know it. One night, we're the only two people left in the office. What happens next?"*

BEST. SEX. EVER.

CONFESSIONS

"The Hottest Sext I've Ever Received Was..."

"I love getting instructions for kink scenes. It builds up what is coming so well in my head. A favorite was a schoolgirl threesome scene where the three of us texted in character for a week leading up to our playdate." **—Natalie, 37**

"My wife and I had been fighting, and she sent me a picture of herself from her office, stripped down to her panties, sitting on her desk. The message just said, 'Let's forget about the argument. Meet me at home in 45 minutes.' I don't think I ever cut out of work so fast." **—Nate, 43**

"A friend with benefits sent an audio recording of him orgasming. That was hot." **—Christi, 24**

"The night of my high school 30th reunion, a woman I was not at all friends with, albeit in a small class of 35 seniors, sent me a picture of herself in the bed of my truck rather exposed...with the caption 'Come and get it.'" **—Edward, 52**

"An ex-boyfriend would snap me pics or videos of him jacking off and cumming in the middle of the night, saying he woke up thinking about me." **—Brian, 39**

TALK DIRTY TO ME

When Do Nudes Come In?

At the start of any (halfway decent) hookup, the sexual tension builds and builds until, *bam*, you're both naked and ready to get it on. Sometimes the same thing happens when you're sexting: Trade enough kinky texts and you might reach a point where you're so turned on, the natural next step is swapping sexy selfies.

At the risk of sounding like your high school sex ed teacher, always assume there's a risk that any naked picture could end up online. We wish it weren't the case, but some people suck, so choose your recipient(s) wisely—and crop out your face, Engle advises. "There is no reason anybody's face needs to be in a nude picture." One more friendly reminder while we're at it: Consent, once again, is a must. Sending someone an out-of-the-blue nude could be considered illegal, depending on how the person interprets it.

Now back to the fun stuff. You get to see someone naked! And show off your own hot bod! Here's what to know about asking for, taking, sending, and storing nudes.

Ask for nudes only if you're prepared to send them in return.
Texting "PLS SEND NUDES"? Yeah, uh, please *don't*. "They're not your personal jack-off material generator," Engle says. Instead, ask if they're down to trade sexy pics.

Get artsy with it.
Show them how much you care by putting some effort into your nudes—i.e., no more down-the-pants snaps from a public bathroom stall. "Make sure you're finding your best lighting," Engle says. "The gym locker room with its disgusting fluorescent lighting is probably not the best

place for your nude photos. Soft lighting is always best." Use your phone's self-timer if it helps you pull off a better pose.

Don't take one shot and hit "send."

"Take a couple and then pick your best one," Engle says. Or better yet, set aside some time for a naked photo shoot where you take a bunch of pics to store on your phone. That way, you won't have to scramble to get a good shot the second your partner asks for one. (It also frees you up to send nudes when you couldn't otherwise take them—like during a subway ride to work.)

Store your nudes on an app.

Speaking of storing sexy selfies on your phone, don't keep 'em on your camera roll, where anyone—think your mom—could accidentally land on them after swiping through your innocent vacation pics. "There are so many apps that are designed for this that are encrypted—you can hide them in a folder," Engle says. Search "encrypted photo storage app" and find one that meets your needs.

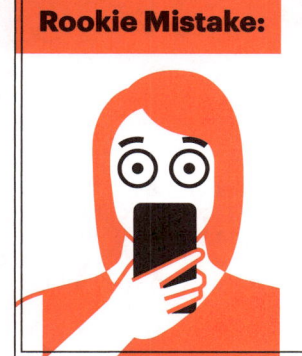

Rookie Mistake:

The *Unsolicited* Dick Pic

You wouldn't flash some hottie you passed on the street, and the same principle applies here. Whether it's an IRL or virtual interaction, ask a partner for permission before you whip out your junk. "People deserve respect," Engle says. "I don't care if this is someone you're talking to on Tinder or somebody you've been dating for five years—this person deserves to be treated like a human being."

TALK DIRTY TO ME

THE BEST POSITIONS FOR...
TAKING A SEXY SELFIE

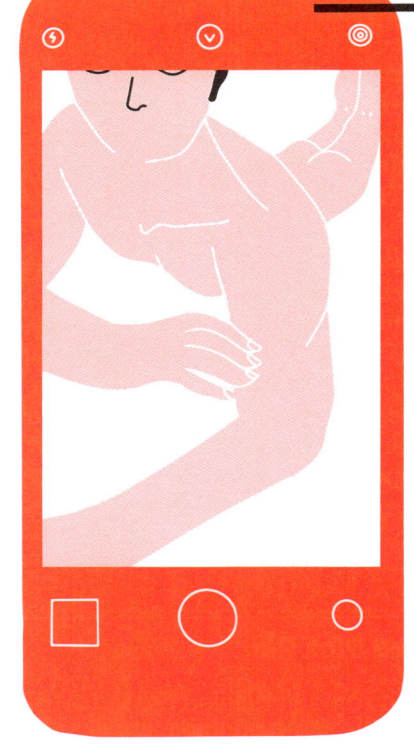

↑ MOUNTAIN VIEW

Lie flat on your stomach and lift your butt (hi, lower back muscles). You'll want to shift the camera slightly to the side so your booty is visible behind your head.

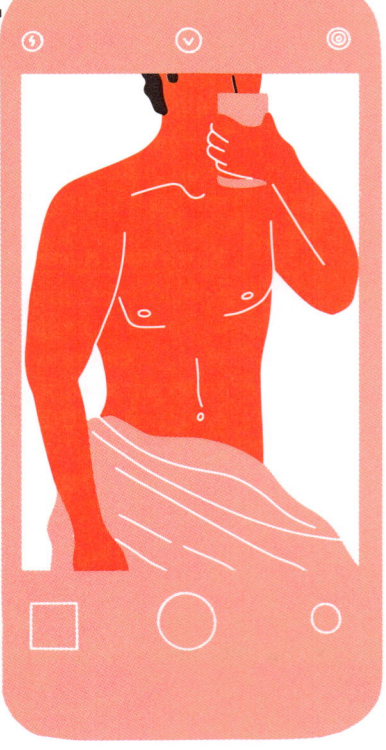

↑ SELF-REFLECTION

Take a selfie in front of the mirror, either with a towel around your waist as a tease or fully in the nude. Just remember to tidy up your bathroom first—you want all eyes on you, not the cluttered mess on the counter.

BEST. SEX. EVER.

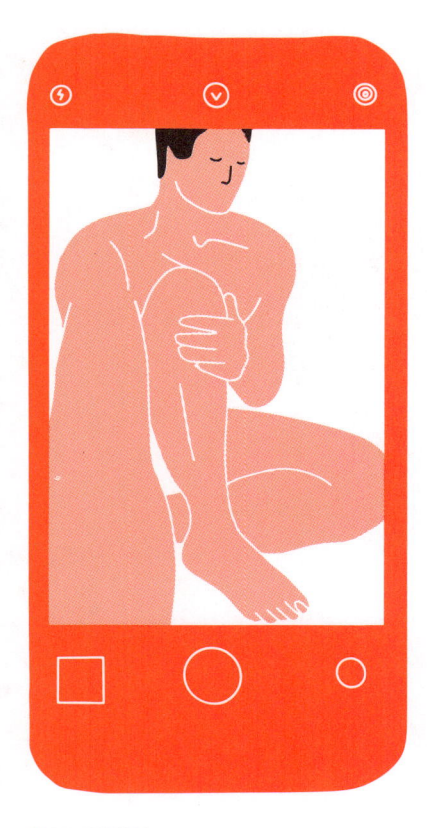

↑ THE TEASE
Get totally naked, but find a way to position yourself so you're covering up your most private bits. It'll leave them hungry for more.

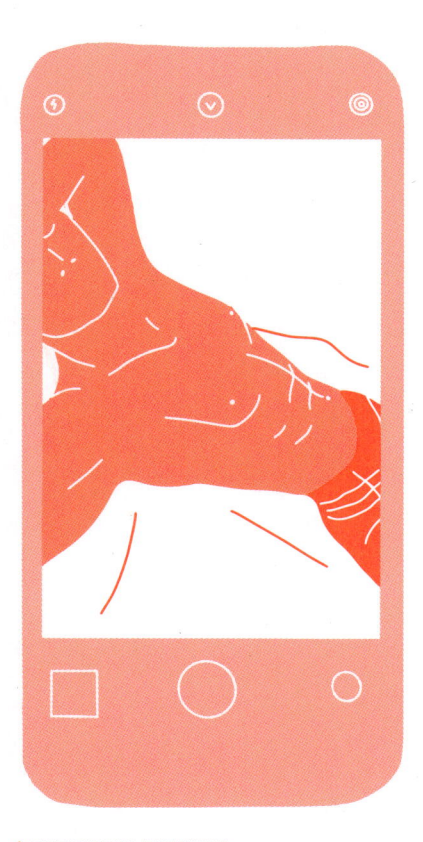

↑ THE BIRD'S-EYE VIEW
Aka "behold the results of my crunch routine." "The downward angle will accentuate your abs," Engle says.

TALK DIRTY TO ME

Now That We're in Bed, What Do I Say?

All right, you're now a pro when it comes to digital dirty talk. Next, we're going to talk about bringing that silver tongue of yours into the bedroom.

We talked about dirty talk stage fright (see page 34), but the truth is, no one's expecting you to transform into a character and deliver a Tony-worthy performance. "It's all about building erotic charge through your voice," Engle says—and there are a bunch of easy ways to do it that don't require a theater degree. Here are a few tips to keep in mind.

Tell a story.

"A lot of dirty talk is storytelling," Engle says. "You can frame it as a sexy dream you had, or maybe it was something you saw in an erotic clip." Just describing the scene (instead of acting it out) can be hot as hell.

Narrate what's literally happening.

If imagination isn't your strong suit, feel free to give a play-by-play of what's happening in the moment. Try talking about...

What you're putting where:

- *"I'm about to put my tongue on that clit."*
- *"I love sliding this butt plug into your ass."*
- *"I'm going to put my dick in your pussy now."*

What you're looking at:

- *"You have the sexiest ass I've ever seen."*
- *"I love seeing how hard you get for me."*
- *"Your tits look amazing right now."*

How something feels:
- *"Your mouth around my cock feels unbelievable."*
- *"I'm going to cum so hard from being inside you."*
- *"I love feeling how wet you get for me."*

Throw in a bunch of descriptive words.

The more adjectives you can add into whatever you're talking about, the better. "The thing that makes dirty talk dirtier is making it more visual," Engle says. Let's take one of the aforementioned examples: "I'm about to put my tongue on that clit." Now let's jack it up to: "I'm about to put my hot, wet tongue on that gorgeous, throbbing clit." "Just add adjectives in there," Engle says, "and you'll see that it suddenly becomes this cyclone of filth."

Try using some of these words:
- *Aching*
- *Amazing*
- *Beautiful*
- *Cute*
- *Gorgeous*
- *Hot*
- *Juicy*
- *Perfect*
- *Sexy*
- *Soft*
- *Sweet*
- *Throbbing*
- *Tight*
- *Unbelievable*
- *Wet*

TALK DIRTY TO ME

BONUS! BUILD YOUR OWN DIRTY TALK

It's time to put your own spin on more sexy scripts from Engle. Fill in the blanks and fire away.

OPTION 1	OPTION 2	OPTION 3
	THE COMPLIMENT:	
I love it when you **VERB** my **ADJECTIVE NOUN**.	You have the most **ADJECTIVE NOUN**.	You're so good at **VERB+ING** my **NOUN**.
	THE ANTICIPATION:	
I'm going to **VERB** your **NOUN** with my **NOUN**.	I'm going to **VERB** all over your/in your **NOUN**.	If you're not good, I'm going to **VERB** all over your/on your **NOUN**.
	THE REQUEST:	
I want to touch your **NOUN** with my **NOUN**.	Will you **VERB** your/my **NOUN**?	I've been naughty/bad. I deserve **FILL IN THE BLANK**.

BEST. SEX. EVER.

SEXPLAIN IT

Dear Sexplain It,

A new sex partner was using a vibrator on herself, and I said, "Be a good girl and play with your toys for Daddy." She frowned and said my comment was creepy. I started apologizing, and she said, "It's fine. It was just weird." We finished having sex, but we weren't in sync like before, and things were tense until I left. She hasn't responded to my texts since then, and I'm afraid it's because of what I said. Is there something I should text her now, and how do I avoid this debacle in the future?

—Failed Dirty Talker

Dear Failed Dirty Talker,

If you've already texted her a few times with no response, my advice is to move along. Your faux pas is an unfortunate reason to end an otherwise blossoming relationship, but as they say, that's the way the cookie crumbles.

If you've texted her just once and she hasn't replied, then I think it's fair for you to reach out *one* final time—but you need to address the elephant in the room. Don't text, "Hey! How was your week?" Acknowledge her feelings and admit you were wrong to assume she was interested in that particular kind of role play without checking first, explains sex and relationship expert Shamyra Howard, L.C.S.W., a member of the *Men's Health* advisory panel: "Let her know that you're committed to showing up differently" if she chooses to hang out with you again. I'm not a fan of long-winded apology texts. I would text her something along the lines of "Hey! I just want to apologize again for what I said during our last hookup. I shouldn't have assumed that you'd be into it. I should have asked first, and I won't make assumptions like this again. I really like you and would like to keep seeing you if you're interested, but if not, I completely understand." You have your answer if she doesn't reply. You move on and are mildly consoled by the most annoying dating advice in existence: There are plenty of fish in the sea.

On to your next question: How do you avoid this predicament in the future? I'm a kinky little bastard, but the first time I have sex with someone I'm really crushing on, I keep things vanilla. I think it can be beneficial to see what your "base level" of sex is: How do you connect *without* toys, role play, and dirty talk? I also think it takes away some of the pressure. If the first time we have sex, I ask to do more of my wild kinks (more on those in Chapter 6), the person I'm dating may feel a little intimidated or turned off. After your first time doing it, *then* you can have a conversation about what kind of dirty talk, role-playing scenarios, and other kinks you're both into. These conversations are only awkward if you make them awkward. If you're smiling and relaxed, your partner will be much more likely to respond in kind.

So, my friend, you messed up, but *barely*. I wouldn't beat yourself up over it. Hopefully she comes around and gives you a second chance, but if not, go ahead and find someone else who really wants to be daddy's little girl. Screw it, I'll be your little girl if you're game.

BEST. SEX. EVER.

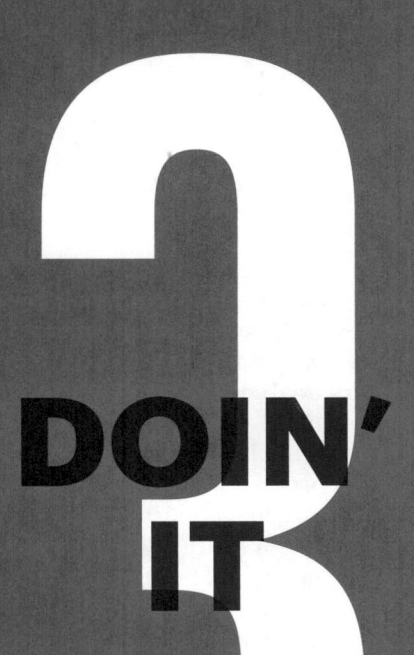

YOUR SEXPERT

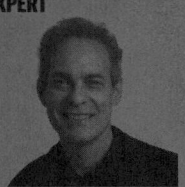

Ian Kerner, Ph.D., L.M.F.T., is a licensed psychotherapist, a nationally recognized sexuality counselor, and the best-selling author of *She Comes First*.

CHAPTER 3

DOIN' IT

Let's roll up our sleeves and get into the mechanics of sex in its myriad forms. (Spoiler: You'll need some lube.)

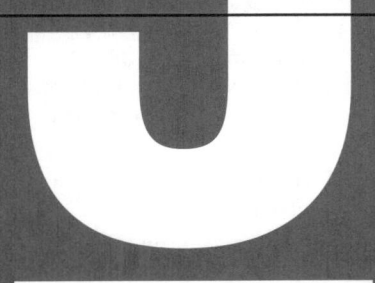

DOIN' IT

Do I Actually Need to Worry About Lasting Longer in Bed?

How come so many cisgender men [meaning their gender identity matches their sex assigned at birth] want to last longer in bed when, in reality, most people on the receiving end of vaginal or anal sex aren't looking for hours of penetration? (Ouch!)
KERNER: I think there are a couple of things. One, all of this is considered a sign of prowess to a guy. He considers it a source of self-esteem. You could almost say that it's a form of sexual narcissism to be able to go as long as you can.

Also, I talk to a lot of couples, and for 95 percent of couples I work with, sex pretty much culminates—or attempts to culminate—in intercourse. And the time leading up to intercourse is anywhere from zero to not much more than ten minutes. So a lot of couples are getting to intercourse within ten minutes, but they still want to connect; they still want to have fun. It also puts a lot of emphasis on intercourse as the main behavior with which to build and sustain arousal.

But there's so much more to sex than the classic framework of a few minutes of foreplay plus intercourse. What's the sexual framework more people *should* be following?
Even though most of us go into sex not thinking about procreating, the way in which we're having sex is still in a very procreative form. Really, we're trying to have sex that brings us closer to somebody—or we're trying to have sex that's recreational, that's fun, that's adventurous, that's whimsical. So if you think about it, intercourse is definitely the best position suited to procreation, but it's not the best

sexual behavior suited to other types of sexual interactions that are relational and recreational.

I think an outercourse-based model, as opposed to an intercourse-based model of sexual expression, is more suited to relational and recreational sex.

What falls under the category of "outercourse"?
First and foremost, I'm talking about taking a clitoral approach to sex. That could be with manual stimulation; it could be oral stimulation; it could be with a sex toy. [Cis] men love outercourse too. There was a study of gay men and the sexual behaviors they engaged in during the last time they had sex, and only 35 percent had anal intercourse—so 65 percent had engaged in other activities that were *not* intercourse-based.

In your experience as a sex therapist, do penis-owners enjoy outercourse as much as vulva-owners do?
I hear from a lot of [cis] men who love oral sex and manual stimulation just as much as they love intercourse. And I hear from many [cis] men who love *giving* oral sex and manually stimulating their partners more than they like intercourse, because it really relieves [them] of so much pressure. To be able to make love with their hands and their mouths and their tongues and a sex toy— it takes all of that pressure off the penis. I'm not against intercourse; I just think it shouldn't be a behavior that overshadows all others.

DOIN' IT

How Can I Up My Oral Game?

We're so glad you asked (and your partner is too). Not only is oral a key component of the outercourse model Kerner talks about, but some people say it's even *more* intimate than intercourse. After all, you're *really* getting up close and personal with another person's vulva, penis, or booty. (See Chapter 5 for everything to know about anilingus.) The best way to please your partner is simple: Ask them what they like. That said, there *are* some oral best practices.

If you're going down on a vulva, wait until your partner's aroused; if they're not, it could hurt or feel ticklish, Kerner says. (The same goes for jumping straight to direct clit stimulation; you might want to head for the labia first.) If you're doing something that's working, stick with it instead of switching up your technique—especially if they're getting close to orgasm. "With cunnilingus, less can be more, and persistence, consistency, and engaging in the right activity at the right time [are key]," Kerner says.

With blowjobs, you also want to start slowly. Tease the penis with your fingers and tongue until your partner's fully erect—then you can suck harder. The wetter, the better; don't be afraid to spit directly onto the penis before and during a BJ. When your partner tells you they're getting close, "apply more pressure at the base and more friction at the head," Kerner says. Keep that stimulation going all the way through their orgasm. (If you'd rather they didn't ejaculate in your mouth, you can switch to just using your hand at the end.)

BEST. SEX. EVER.

And you can always try getting your hands or a toy involved. Lots of folks enjoy receiving external clitoral or penile stimulation while their partner also touches their vagina, testicles, perineum, or anus. There are so many possible combos: Think licking your partner's clit while you use a dildo in their vagina or sucking your partner's penis with one hand wrapped around their shaft and the other massaging their perineum.

Pro Tip: ➡ Bring Balls Into the BJ

When giving blowjobs, a lot of people focus solely on the head and shaft of the penis. Yes, those two areas should be primary focuses, but they shouldn't be the only things you're stimulating when you're going down on your partner. "While going down, you can cup the balls," Kerner says. Some guys even like to have their testicles sucked on lightly. (If you pull their testicles too far down or away from their body, it can be painful, so be careful.)

DOIN' IT

THE BEST POSITIONS FOR...
ORAL SEX ON A VULVA

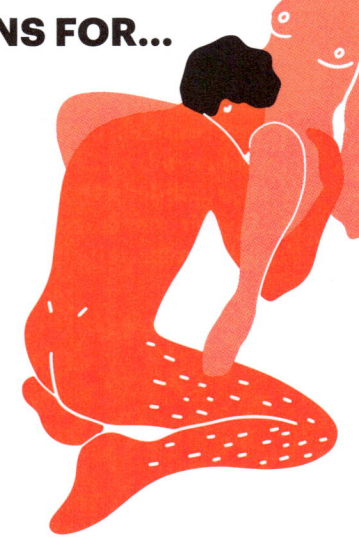

PUT YOUR LEG IN THE AIR (LIKE YOU JUST DON'T CARE) ↓

Many people with a vulva find they're more sensitive on one side of the clitoris, and this is the perfect sex position to make the most of that heightened sensitivity. The receiver lies on the bed with one leg in the air while the giver kneels on the floor. (Note: The receiver should raise the leg corresponding to the sensitive side of the clitoris—it'll help expose the area to the giver's tongue.)

↑ HEIR TO THE THRONE

This position is great for playing with power dynamics. The receiving partner gets to feel like royalty as they perch on a throne (or, you know, an ottoman or chair) while the giver kneels on the floor.

BEST. SEX. EVER.

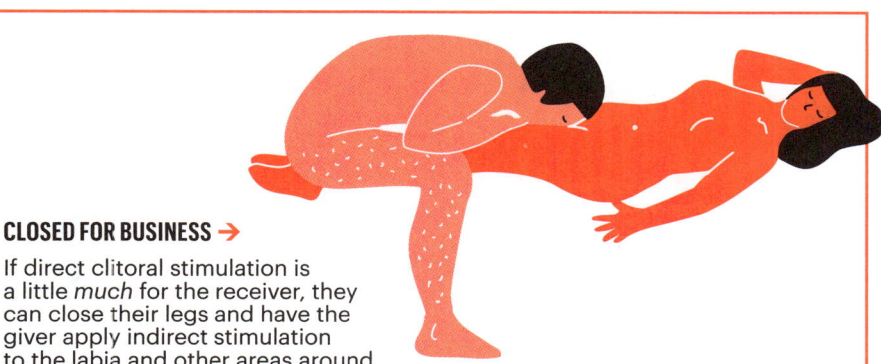

CLOSED FOR BUSINESS →

If direct clitoral stimulation is a little *much* for the receiver, they can close their legs and have the giver apply indirect stimulation to the labia and other areas around the clit. You could warm up in this position before transitioning into something more intense, or just stay here for the duration!

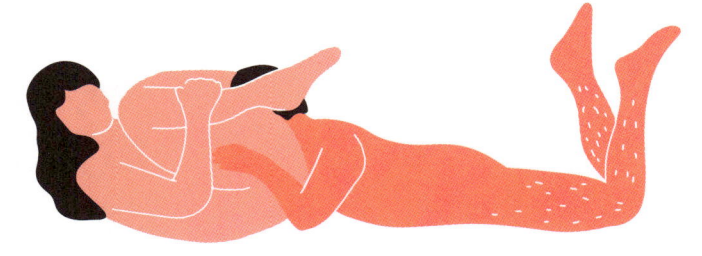

↖ THE ROLY-POLY

This position is essentially an all-access pass to the receiver's vulva and anus, if rimming is on the menu. (See page 110!)

THE KIVIN METHOD ↘

This is basically sideways cunnilingus, and some people with a vulva say it helps them achieve orgasm faster. To make it feel even better, the giver can use their hand to apply pressure to the receiver's taint.

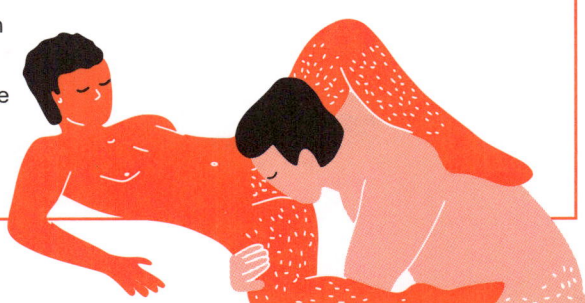

53

DOIN' IT

THE BEST POSITIONS FOR...
BLOWJOBS

↓ SIDEWAYS 69
For when the OG 69 gets old. Plus, less neck strain.

THE FACE-SITTER ↑
This one makes it easy to play with dominant and submissive roles. And it's great for deep-throating—if that's something both of you are into.

HUMP AND BLOW →
With one leg wrapped around the giver, the receiver can actually thrust into their partner in this position. (Obviously, if you're the receiver, make sure your partner is cool with said thrusting before you go to town.)

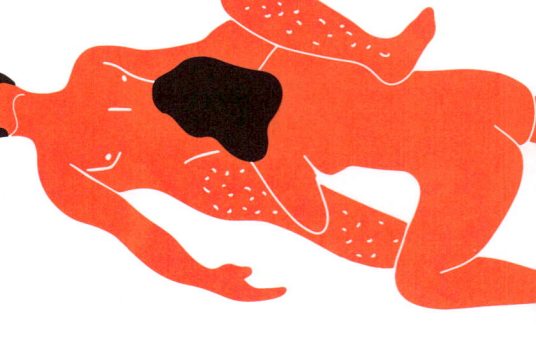

BEST. SEX. EVER.

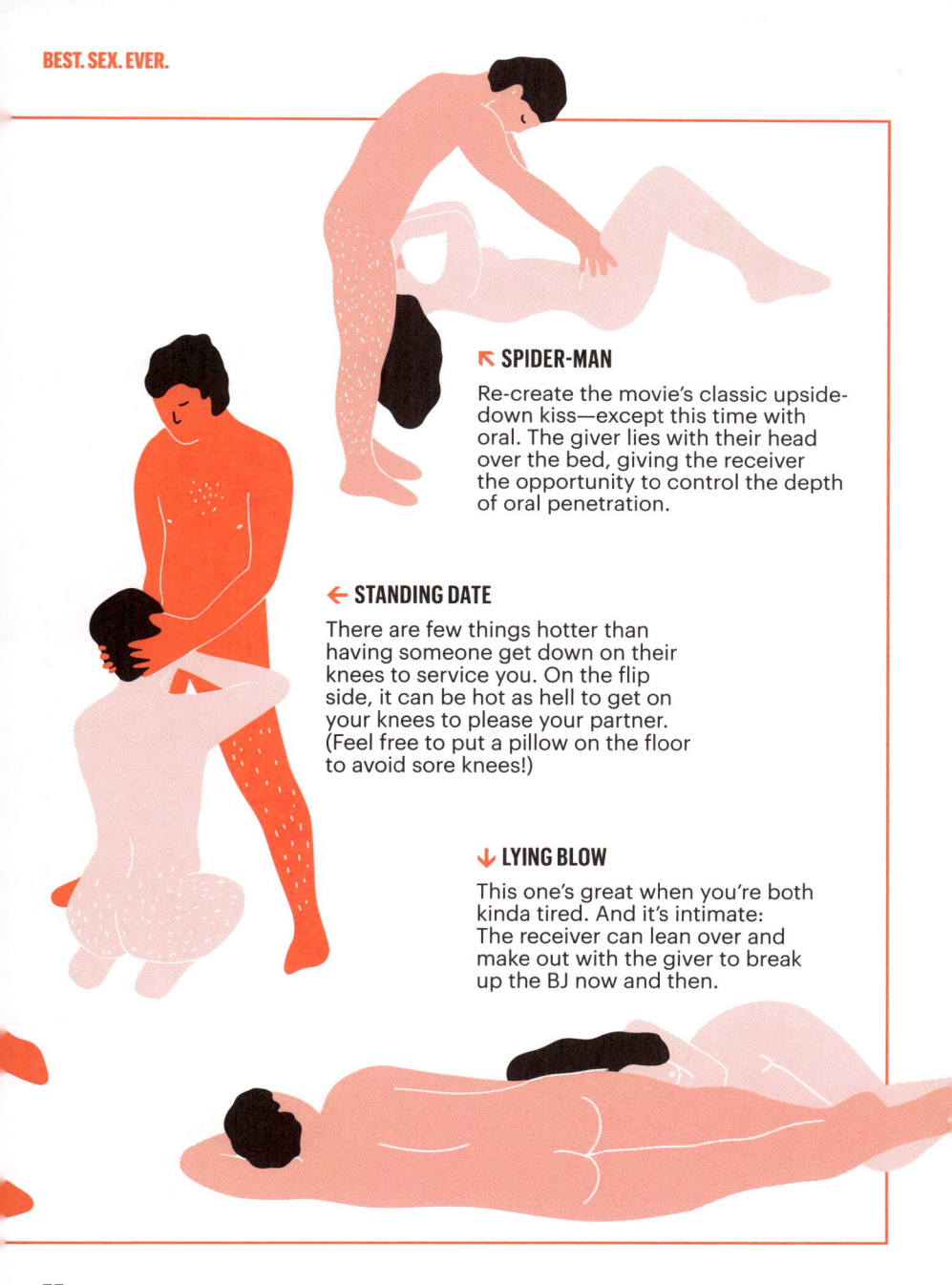

↖ SPIDER-MAN

Re-create the movie's classic upside-down kiss—except this time with oral. The giver lies with their head over the bed, giving the receiver the opportunity to control the depth of oral penetration.

← STANDING DATE

There are few things hotter than having someone get down on their knees to service you. On the flip side, it can be hot as hell to get on your knees to please your partner. (Feel free to put a pillow on the floor to avoid sore knees!)

↓ LYING BLOW

This one's great when you're both kinda tired. And it's intimate: The receiver can lean over and make out with the giver to break up the BJ now and then.

DOIN' IT

THE BEST _____ EVER

The Best Oral Sex I've Ever Received

"I will always remember the guy who deep-throated me for the first time. No one else had managed it before then, but he swallowed me whole, and my mind was just blown at how amazing it felt to be down someone's throat like that." **—Curtis, 38**

"In a threesome with my wife and her friend when they both went down on me at the same time. They took turns swapping between my shaft and my balls." **—Nate, 43**

"69ing with a former boyfriend. I love the concept of trying to show off for one another and the aspect of competition to make one another cum." **—Gregg, 30**

"Getting a BJ on a walking trail in the middle of the day. The guy kissed the back of my knees, which was weird but kinda hot." **—Slade, 32**

"When my fiancée was sucking on my cock and then she put in a vibrator to milk my prostate." **—Willie, 36**

"He was on his knees, butt plug in, when I opened the door, and [he] gave me the best BJ ever. I was face-fucking him, all sweaty after the gym." **—Rudy, 32**

BEST. SEX. EVER.

How Do I Find a Condom That Doesn't Suck?

If you use 'em correctly, condoms are highly effective at preventing unwanted pregnancy and many sexually transmitted infections (STIs), yet recent data shows that condom use is declining in the United States while STI rates continue to rise. (While we're on the topic of STIs: Get tested! Talk to your doctor about the testing types and frequency that best fit your life.)

There are a variety of reasons penis-owners aren't using rubbers, including the country's sorry state of sex education and the fact that we rarely (if ever) see them in porn. But one of the most common excuses? They just don't feel good—which is wrong for a number of reasons. "Condoms don't have to be the enemy of pleasure," Kerner says. "They can actually be an accessory to pleasure."

There are condoms that are ridged, that are super-duper thin, that have numbing agents in them to help with premature ejaculation. It might take some trial and error to find the condom that works best for you and your partner. "You have to find the right texture, the right size, the right feel overall," Kerner says. Remember, if your penis feels like it's being strangled, the condom is probably too small (and runs the risk of breaking during sex); if your penis feels like it's going to slip out, the condom is probably too big.

Condoms are colloquially known as "rubbers," but they're made from other materials too. *Latex*—i.e., the rubber variety—is the most commonly sold option, although some folks can't use them due to a latex allergy. That's where condoms made from *polyisoprene* (synthetic rubber) and *polyurethane* (ultra-thin, flexible plastic) might come in handy. Another alternative is the *lambskin* condom, made from a part of a lamb's large intestine. Some people say lambskin condoms feel the most natural, but remember: They prevent only pregnancy—not STIs.

Another reason some people shy away from condom use? They're stressed about it messing with their erection, according to Kerner. "A lot of [cis] men really worry that in the transition of putting on a condom—or once the condom is on—they're going to lose their erection," he says. "And then, worrying about it, it starts to become a self-fulfilling prophecy." (For tips on kicking performance anxiety's ass, check out page 78.)

Finally, there's the perceived awkwardness factor. Some men worry that pausing to put on a rubber will "take them out of the moment," Kerner says. If that's been the case for you, it might be a sign that your whole hook-up could use more sexual tension. "If you're really into the sex and you're really simmering that arousal, then taking 30 seconds to put on a condom is nothing," Kerner says. "In fact, it's going to build anticipation."

Will wearing a condom feel *exactly* like not wearing one? No! We're not going to pretend the experiences are 100 percent interchangeable.

But if sex feels "ruined" because of a *slightly* different sensation on your peen, you might need to alter your approach to sex. "If you're so focused on a condom not feeling good, I'm sorry, you're just too focused on your penis," Kerner says. "You're telling me, in a way, that only your penis is at the heart of arousal; you're telling me your mind is not aroused and other parts of your body might not be aroused.

"You're not fully sensitized, because sex is not just a penis-based experience—it's really a full-body, mind-based experience."

BEST. SEX. EVER.

Pro Tip: ➡ Wear a Condom

While there isn't a risk of pregnancy when having anal sex, there is still a risk of STIs. Gonorrhea, syphilis, chlamydia, HSV (herpes), HPV, and HIV can all be spread through anal sex, and condoms are the best way to prevent contracting and spreading these STIs. Luckily, gonorrhea, syphilis, and chlamydia are all treatable with antibiotics. If you're having penetrative sex often and you aren't consistent with your condom use, then you should consider taking PrEP (pre-exposure prophylaxis) to mitigate the risk of HIV.

At the time of writing there are currently two FDA-approved antiretroviral medications, Truvada and Descovy, which can be taken as a means of PrEP. These daily medications decrease the likelihood of acquiring HIV through sex by about 99 percent.

DOIN' IT

Do I Need to Use Lube?

We'll answer with a question: Do you like it when sex is smooth and wet, or do you prefer a dry, friction-heavy experience? We're gonna go ahead and assume you picked the first option. Listen, it'd be great if everyone's junk got all slippery on its own, but that's just not how bodies work. The vagina doesn't always self-lubricate, and the anus *never* does. No matter what kind of sex you're having, lube can make it smoother (translation: hotter).

We'll admit that the word *lube* is decidedly unsexy. But using it in the heat of the moment doesn't have to be. Kerner recommends reaching for it as you tell your partner how sexy they are or even working it into an erotic massage. (Use massage oil on their back and lube on their junk.) "It's not about making the lube *itself* sexy," Kerner says. "It's about just incorporating it into how you are sexually appreciating and getting turned on by your partner."

Some trans men on hormones see a decrease in natural lubrication as it can be a potential side effect of taking testosterone, Pitagora says. "The key for trans men who do enjoy receiving penetration but are experiencing pain is to use lubrication generously," they add. So no matter your gender, sexual orientation, or what kind of sex you're having, lube can make it smoother (translation: hotter).

There are four main kinds of lube, each with its own pros and cons:

Water-based lube doesn't get sticky, is easy to wash off, and won't stain the sheets, but it dries out quickly; use it for any kind of sex, as long as you're down to reapply often.

Silicone-based lube is thicker, longer-lasting, and great for penetration and all kinds of anal activity, although it can feel a little too sticky, so consider a *water-silicone hybrid lube* if you want the best of both worlds. (Also, careful if you're pairing silicone lube with silicone sex toys—it can break down your toys over time.)

Finally, there's *oil-based lube*, best saved for external activities like massages; it erodes latex condoms and can irritate the vagina, making it a poor choice for any kind of penetration.

Rookie Mistake: **Using _Spit_ Instead of _Lube_**

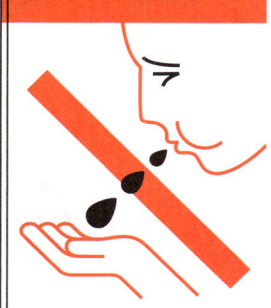

But they do it all the time in porn! Yeah, well, porn is fake, but physical discomfort is real. "If you're going down on someone, saliva can be a decent lubricant, but for any kind of real penetration, it just doesn't work," Kerner says. "You're going to need something that's silicone-based, that is just more slippery and doesn't dry up as quickly." (And while water-based lube takes some reapplying, it *still* lasts longer than spit, FYI.)

DOIN' IT

THE BEST POSITIONS FOR...
APPRECIATING THE CLASSICS

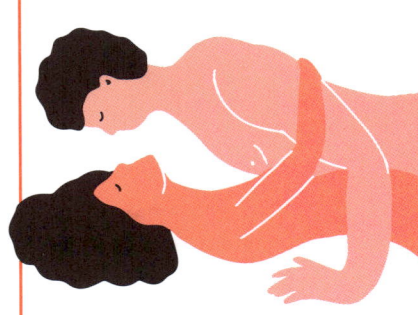

MISSIONARY ↗

Lie face-to-face with the penetrating partner on top and the receiving partner on their back. Sure, it's "traditional," but there's also a lot to love about missionary, like the intimacy of being close and the opportunity for making out.

↓ COWGIRL

The partner on top can maximize their pleasure by controlling the depth and speed of penetration. Introduce a vibrator for some clitoral action on top of the G-spot and cervical stimulation.

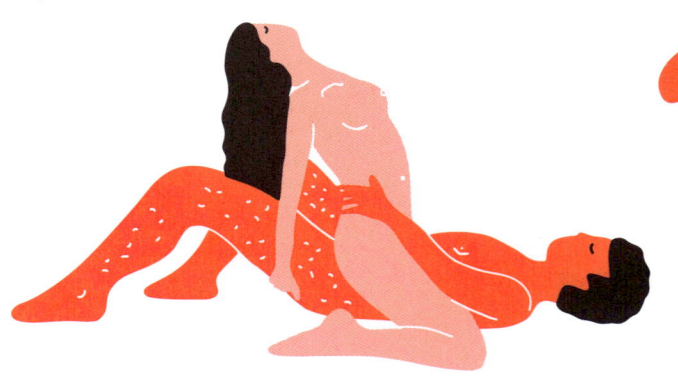

BEST. SEX. EVER.

69 →

On the one hand, it's super sexy *and* super productive. On the other hand, some people find it hard to focus on giving and receiving at the same time.

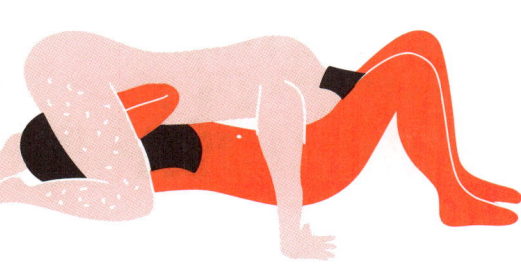

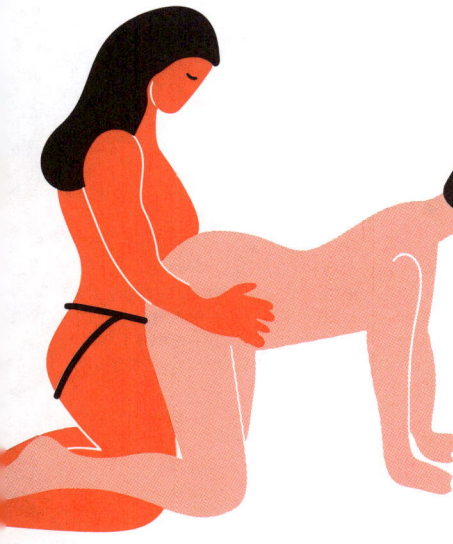

← DOGGY STYLE

This one's great for vaginal and anal intercourse—not to mention going *deep*. The penetrating partner can feel free to reach around to offer some finger-based (or sex-toy-enhanced) action too.

SPOONING →

You both lie on your sides facing the same way, the penetrating partner entering the receiving partner from behind. It's basically cuddling, with more orgasms.

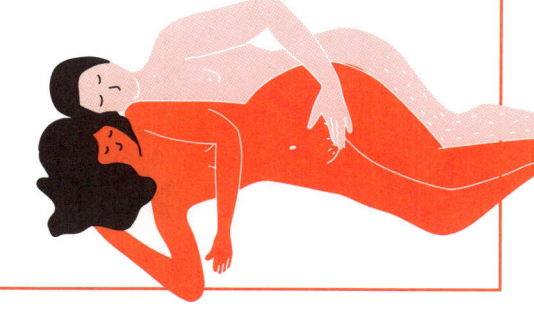

DOIN' IT

THE BEST POSITIONS FOR...
MAKING SEX WORK FOR YOUR BODY

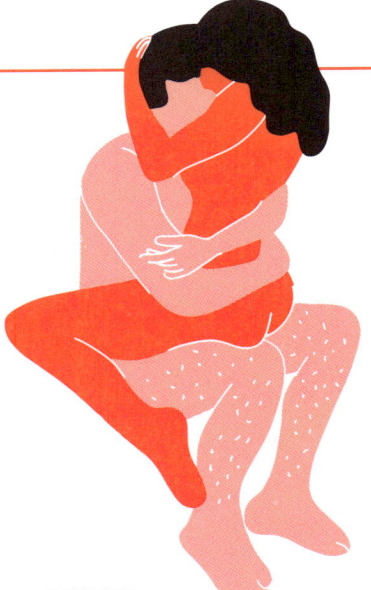

FACE-OFF ↗

If the giving partner has pain or restricted mobility, Kerner recommends bringing in supportive furniture. "It can be one partner sitting on a chair with the support they need and a partner on top of them," he says.

↖ HOT SEAT

It's the same idea as the face-off but with the receiving partner facing away. (Think of it as "doggy in a chair," Kerner says.)

BEST. SEX. EVER.

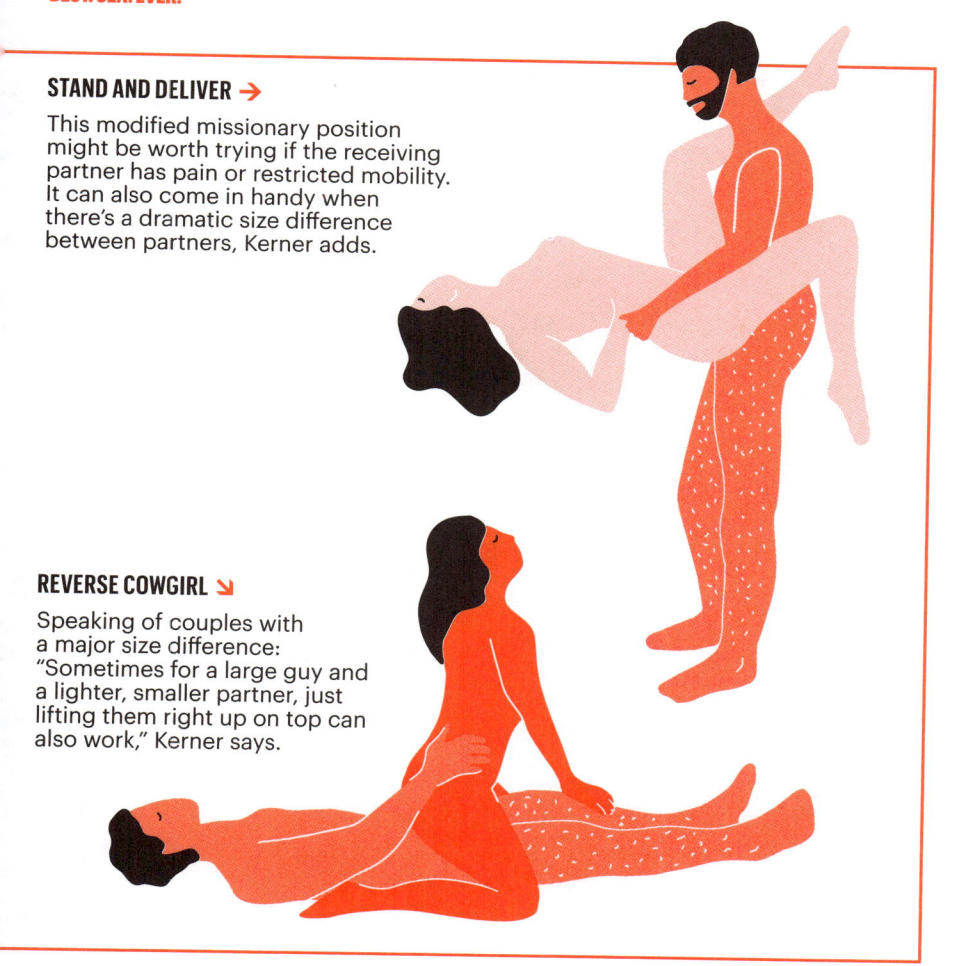

STAND AND DELIVER →

This modified missionary position might be worth trying if the receiving partner has pain or restricted mobility. It can also come in handy when there's a dramatic size difference between partners, Kerner adds.

REVERSE COWGIRL ↘

Speaking of couples with a major size difference: "Sometimes for a large guy and a lighter, smaller partner, just lifting them right up on top can also work," Kerner says.

Pro Tip: ➡ Use the Pelvis Pillow

If you and your partner can't get your junk to line up *juuust* right, consider putting a pillow—either a specially designed sex pillow or any old sturdy cushion—under the receiving partner's pelvis to prop them up. (If the receiving partner has a vulva, playing with a pillow can also unlock new and satisfying angles.)

DOIN' IT

What if My Partner Prefers a Sex Toy to Me?

Let's say a specific kind of dirty talk really got your partner off. Would you feel somehow threatened by those erotic words? Hell no! You'd probably be like, "I just discovered this amazing new sex tool, and I can't wait to use it again!" The same goes for using sex toys. Maybe because some of them resemble body parts (think a dildo) and go places body parts go, it's easier to feel like you're competing with them—but you're not. Sure, they can do things a human body can't do, such as vibrate, pulse, or provide hours of suction, but that's all the more reason you should want them on your team!

Vibrators, dildos, cock rings, butt plugs, prostate massagers, and other toys can help you expand your sexual skills, experience pleasure in new ways, and bring an overall sense of excitement to your bedroom routine. For people with a vulva, sex toys—specifically clitoral vibrators—can also increase the odds of climaxing. (See page 174 for more on how the vast majority of vulva-owners require clitoral stimulation to reach orgasm.) "We talk a lot about the orgasm gap," says Kerner, referring to the fact that heterosexual cis women are far less likely to orgasm during sex than heterosexual cis men. "A lot of that has to do with relying on intercourse alone, as opposed to intercourse plus some form of clitoral stimulation."

"More and more couples are incorporating sex toys and vibration into their sex play because they're mutually pleasurable, but they also allow a lot of positions to generate pleasure," he adds. Think reaching around during doggy style to hold a bullet vibrator on your partner's clit or having them play with a vibe while they lie on their back in the aforementioned stand and deliver position (page 65 for a refresher).

There are a gazillion ways to use sex toys as a couple. Here are a few ideas to inspire you:

- Massage your partner's G-spot with a dildo or wand while you lick their clitoris. (See: the Venus butterfly position on page 177.)
- Have your partner hold a vibrator to their clit during vaginal or anal penetration.
- Gradually pull anal beads out of your partner's ass while you give them a blowjob.
- Use a prostate massager on yourself while your partner jerks you off—or vice versa.
- Pop in a butt plug or slide on a vibrating cock ring (or why not both?) before you top your partner during anal sex.
- Tie up your partner and tease them by holding a vibrator to different erogenous zones.
- And pegging. Obviously. (See page 69.)

Pro Tip: ➡ How to Find Gender-Affirming Sex Toys

Most sex toy companies are stuck in the past. They use language assuming that all men have penises/all women have vaginas, and all people care about is penetrative sex. This simply isn't true and can make the process of buying a sex toy uncomfortable and exclusionary for trans and nonbinary folks. Luckily, "there are sex toy companies that are run by queer and/or trans people, so those sex toys are usually described using language that isn't stuck in a heteronormative gender binary," Pitagora says. The best way to find them is to simply Google "transgender sex toys."

DOIN' IT

THE BUYER$ GUIDE TO...
SEX TOYS TO USE AS A COUPLE

COCK RINGS are bands that you put around your penis. (Some products have two rings: one to place over the base of your penis and the other to place around your testicles.) Some are sturdy and made of metal, whereas others are flexible and made from silicone. And many vibrate, meaning your partner can reap the benefit too.

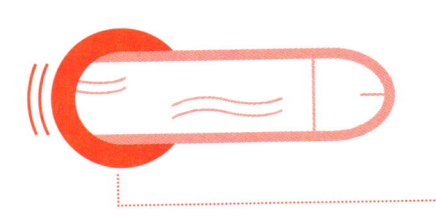

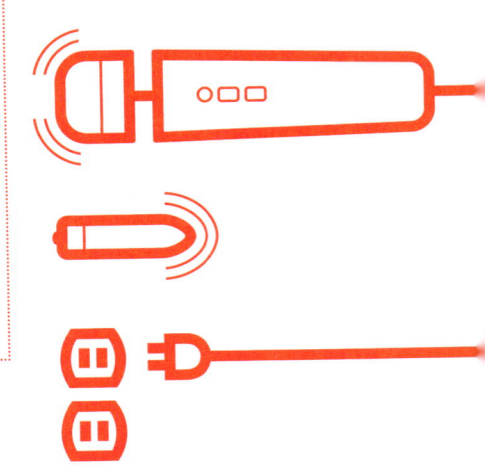

We tend to associate sex toys with masturbation—you know, something you drag outta the bedside drawer whenever a flesh-and-blood partner isn't available. But these toys can also work wonders for all kinds of partnered sex.

BEST. SEX. EVER.

CLITORAL VIBRATORS come in many shapes and sizes, from the finger-size battery-operated bullet vibrators to the forearm-size plug-in Magic Wands. There are even clitoral suction vibrators that mimic the feeling of someone sucking on your clit. Use these toys to make any vaginal intercourse position more pleasurable for the receiver.

PROSTATE MASSAGERS are vibrating toys that go up the anus to stimulate the prostate, a walnut-size gland that's jam-packed with nerve endings (almost as many as the clitoris). Some are hands-free, meaning you can wear 'em during intercourse.

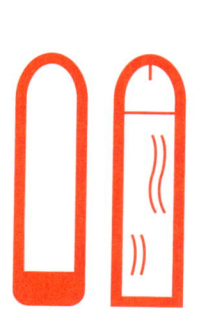

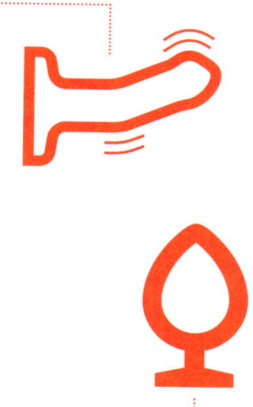

DILDOS are non-vibrating phallic-shaped toys designed for penetration. Some look exactly like a real penis, complete with human skin tones and veins, whereas others are more abstract. One way to use a dildo is *pegging*, i.e., when someone wears a dildo to anally penetrate their partner. (Remember: Any time a toy is going in a butt, it needs to have a flared base—otherwise it could get stuck up there, and no one wants that.)

BUTT PLUGS are non-vibrating toys that sit in your anus and deliver a satisfying feeling of "fullness." You can wear one during all kinds of sexy play.

DOIN' IT

SEXPLAIN IT

Dear Sexplain It,

I'm a 44-year-old man who's never cum from getting head, and it really wasn't all that big of a deal to me—until a few months ago when my second wife and I split. I got together with this one woman, and she was amazing at it. She made me cum in less than a minute.

My question is, how do I go about getting more blowjobs from women? Is it something you just ask for? Is it something where I sorta pull it out and insinuate it? I asked a buddy who is extremely experienced with women, and even he said he didn't have a real answer. In his experience, he said some women just really like to do it and you don't have to do much at all to get them to do it on their own. I feel weird about asking the current woman I'm dating, "Hey, can I have a blowjob?" or whipping it out and saying, "Here you go!" And I don't want to just wait until foreplay and cum from that and then not be able to perform. How is this supposed to work?

—Just Wants Head

Dear Just Wants Head,

First, I just want to say how excited I am for you. Welcome to the enormous club of people who like to have their penis sucked!

The question of how to ask for a BJ pops up in my inbox frequently, so you're not alone. I would like to start by explaining how *not* to ask for a BJ. Do not:

- *"Sorta pull it out and insinuate it." Your penis is not a worm at the end of a hook.*
- *Say, "Here you go!" Your penis is not a holiday gift.*
- *You didn't suggest this, but I'd also like to preemptively caution against the "head push," where you guide their head down to your dick. That's an asshole move. (If you are dating someone and have that dynamic, fine, but don't with someone new who's never given you a BJ.)*

So how do you ask? By having a conversation outside the bedroom about both of your sexual desires. For example, the next time you're having dinner, say, "Hey, I have a fun question for you: What are some sexual things that really turn you on?" After your partner shares her desires, you can talk about yours—including that you love receiving oral. If you express that desire, she'll go into your next hookup knowing it's something you'd enjoy.

That said, there *is* a scenario where she says, "Oh, I really don't like giving head." To learn exactly how to respond to this, I reached out to Rachel Wright, M.A., L.M.F.T., licensed psychotherapist and sex educator. She says that in this situation, "you can kindly ask what they don't like about giving oral sex. Get as much information as you can." The goal here isn't to change your partner's

DOIN' IT

mind if it's a hard limit but rather to see if there's a simple solution to her oral sex aversion. "I've had clients who don't like giving oral because they don't like how sweaty and smelly their partner's penis is," Wright says. In that case, the fix is easy: You shower first. (Honestly, this is good BJ etiquette for everyone.)

Now on to the second part of your question, re: ejaculating from a BJ and then not being able to perform during penetrative sex. Just Wants Head, you need to abandon this idea that there's a strict order to sex. Sex is a lawless land. Let the chaos reign! You can have all kinds of sex before *finishing* with a blowjob, if that's something she's into. Or try this: Start with a BJ. Then go down on your partner for a good long time. Then once you're ready to go again, have P-in-V sex.

"Sex is not linear. It's not a race. Sex is a meaningful act of pleasure," Wright says. Amen.

BEST. SEX. EVER.

YOUR SEXPERT

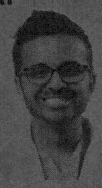

Jamin Brahmbhatt, M.D., is a codirector at the PUR Clinic in Clermont, Florida, which specializes in urology and men's health.

WHAT'S UP WITH MY JUNK?

Dicks can be finicky. Sometimes you can't get things started, and sometimes you finish way too quickly. Then there's the stressful question: Am I big enough? You're not alone in these concerns.

CHAPTER

WHAT'S UP WITH MY JUNK?

Why Doesn't My Penis Work the Way I Want?

There's this idea that if you're under 40, your penis works perfectly all the time. You have no erectile dysfunction and you can always ejaculate. Is this true?
BRAHMBHATT: No, that's absolutely not the case. I've seen teens as young as 17 with erectile dysfunction issues and penis sensitivity issues. It's actually quite common in young [cis] men.

Where does this myth that ED affects only older men with a penis come from?
Well, after 40, [cis] men can start to see a decline in testosterone, which [they] equate with erection issues. So that's where that number comes from. But also, marketing by ED medications like Viagra and Cialis really targeted the baby boomer generation when they first came out because this generation has more problems that cause ED [like arterial plaque buildup, diabetes, obesity, alcoholism, etc.]. So in the psyche of young [cis] men, especially millennials, it's thought of as an older problem. This is not a problem based on age. It can happen anytime.

However, for young cis men, ED has less to do with the body aging and more to do with being nervous. Why is that?

It's hard to differentiate the two. The psychological interacts with the physiological, but yes, the pendulum does shift and it becomes more physiological as you get older since plaque naturally builds up in blood vessels and nerve damage is more common from things like diabetes, multiple sclerosis, and spinal cord and nerve injuries. But there are plenty of young [cis] men also coming in unaware that they have diabetes or very high blood pressure.

When should you see a doctor if you're struggling with ED?

You can honestly go and see a urologist anytime you feel you are having issues in the bedroom. However, here's the problem with that approach: There is a shortage of urologists across the country, so it may take some time to see someone. The good news is that basic ED issues can be managed by your primary care doctor. You can get your labs and testing done there [which will test for heart disease, diabetes, and low testosterone, among other potential causes]. There are also several online clinics offering evaluations for ED. Help is everywhere—you just have to be willing to get it!

WHAT'S UP WITH MY JUNK?

Where Does Performance Anxiety Come From?

Sometimes when our dicks don't work the way we want them to, it's because we get too in our heads. Right as we begin to have sex, we begin to worry: *What if I can't please them? What if I'm not big enough? What if they think my body is disgusting?* These negative, anxiety-inducing thoughts inhibit our ability to perform—either we can't get an erection or we can't maintain an erection or we ejaculate *too* quickly. This is called sexual performance anxiety, and it happens to the best of us.

There are countless reasons for performance anxiety, and they're all interconnected, but Brahmbhatt breaks them down into four distinct categories.

1. Stress

"The number one cause of performance anxiety is stress," Brahmbhatt says. The cause of stress can take many forms. "Some guys who watch a lot of adult entertainment get anxious because they're afraid they're not going to be able to perform like porn stars," he says. This spirals into thinking that they're not going to be able to please their partner.

Then there's simply the stress and anxiety "that comes when transitioning from masturbation to having intercourse," Brahmbhatt says. When you're masturbating by yourself, there's no pressure, but when you're with a partner, you worry about how your body looks, if you're going to be able to satisfy your partner, and so much more. But you could also just be stressed out from work or moving homes or any number of regular stressors. These stressors impede your ability to perform because instead of focusing on (and connecting to) the naked body in front of you, you're thinking about something else, such as your tone in an email you sent to your boss.

2. Alcohol and Drug Dependence

"I see a lot of guys who come in with ED when they have a dependence on alcohol, marijuana, or another substance," Brahmbhatt says. All these things can inhibit an ability to get and maintain an erection, but some guys are too nervous to hook up with partners *without* them, so it becomes a bit of a catch-22.

3. Relationship Problems

"If you've cheated, you may feel guilty and then have trouble getting it up with your partner," Brahmbhatt says. Conversely, if you think your partner is cheating, that could inhibit your ability to perform.

If you're in an unhealthy relationship where your partner is verbally, emotionally, or physically abusive, you also might struggle to perform. But it doesn't have to be that serious. It could be that you two have been arguing a little more than usual, so your body isn't quite feeling it. Your penis, in a weird way, knows you better than you do. If something is off, unhealthy, or even dangerous, it's not going to get erect.

4. Religious or Societal Sex Negativity

If you were brought up in a religious household that says it's not okay to have premarital sex, sex for pleasure, or sex with a person of the same gender, "then you're going to experience a lot of guilt when you have sex," Brahmbhatt says. One of the quickest ways to kill a boner? Feeling guilty about doing it.

So How Do I Deal With Performance Anxiety?

Once you can label what's causing your performance anxiety, it's a lot easier to attack the issue. For example, if you're struggling with alcohol dependence, well, then you should explore steps to treat the problem. If you have religious shame, you need to get into therapy ASAP. If you can't get it up because you cheated, you might need to have a serious talk with your partner about your act of infidelity.

However, sometimes it's difficult to know the root of the problem, or solving the case can take years, or you have some anxiety about your ability to perform that isn't that deep. You're just nervous because sex is a little bit nerve-racking.

"That's when Viagra or Cialis comes into play," Brahmbhatt says. Viagra and Cialis are two prescription medications in the class of phosphodiesterase 5 (PDE5) inhibitors. They work by relaxing muscles in blood vessel walls to help increase blood flow to the penis, making it easier to get and maintain an erection.

It has never been simpler to get prescribed Viagra now that it's generic. You can do so online on health care sites like Hims and Roman. It takes all of 15 minutes. Now if for whatever reason you can't take a PDE5 inhibitor (maybe because of other meds you're on) or you notice it doesn't have an effect, that's when it gets trickier, and you should consult with your primary care doctor to see what they recommend.

BEST. SEX. EVER.

What Are the Medical Reasons for ED?

While anxiety and stress are often the reasons for erectile dysfunction, especially in younger men, there may be an underlying medical condition causing your willy to stay soft. In that case, your ED may be a result of something more serious. If you're struggling with ED and it doesn't seem like it's anxiety-based, you should see a urologist.

It could be an indicator that you have:

Diabetes

"It's not uncommon for men with ED to have undiagnosed diabetes or juvenile type 1 diabetes," Brahmbhatt says. It's estimated that between 35 and 75 percent of cis men with diabetes experience at least some degree of ED during their lifetime. They are also likely to develop ED ten to 15 years earlier than cis men without diabetes.

High Blood Pressure

High blood pressure is yet another factor that can cause ED. Luckily, it's easy to know if you have high blood pressure since it's taken every time you step into your doctor's office. From there, you can work with your primary care doctor to lower your blood pressure and get those hard erections back.

Heart Disease

"Heart disease can alter the blood flow into your penis due to changes that occur inside the lining of the blood vessels [endothelium]," Brahmbhatt says. The endothelial dysfunction then causes inadequate blood supply to the heart and impaired blood flow to the penis.

WHAT'S UP WITH MY JUNK?

Low Testosterone

"Low T does not cause ED directly," Brahmbhatt explains. "But testosterone is vital for sexual libido." If your drive is down, then you are going to have a hard time getting erect because you are just not excited enough to want to do it.

Obesity

"Obesity is known to bring about diabetes, high blood pressure, and high cholesterol," Brahmbhatt says. "All of these medical conditions can alter the blood flow into and out of the penis."

Pro Tip: ➡ *Whiskey Dick* Is Real. Here's How to Avoid It.

Whiskey may make you feel wild and rambunctious, but alas, whiskey and all alcohol are depressants, which decrease blood flow to the penis. That's why all alcohol can cause ED. (Don't let the name fool you. It could just as easily have been called *martini dick* or *mezcal dick*.) The good news is that it typically takes a moderate amount of alcohol to get whiskey dick. One or two drinks and you should be fine. Some penis-owners can have as many as six drinks and not be affected. So you'll have to experiment with what the max is for you, and if you think you're going to get lucky, keep it below that number.

BEST. SEX. EVER.

How Can I Last Longer in Bed?

In a widely quoted study in *The Journal of Sexual Medicine*, researchers had 500 heterosexual couples use stopwatches to measure the time between vaginal penetration and male ejaculation over four weeks of sex sessions. The overall median time was 5.4 minutes, or less than it takes to boil four cups of water. Clearly, this is not a lot of time, especially when you think of how the average woman with a vulva takes 13.41 minutes to orgasm, according to another study published in *The Journal of Sexual Medicine*. So how do you last longer in bed, especially when you're *really* damn turned on?

Luckily, there are various short-term and long-term solutions to keep you pumping away for longer.

Strengthen your pelvic-floor muscles.

You've likely heard of Kegels or Kegel exercises, where you train the pubococcygeal (PC) muscles of your pelvic floor through a series of contraction and release exercises. To understand what these muscles feel like when they're fired up, try cutting off the flow of urine the next time you're peeing. After you cut it off, let it flow, then cut it off again, then let it flow again.

For help isolating those PC muscles, try standing in front of a mirror and then lifting your testicles without the help of your hands. Imagine raising your nuts to your guts or shortening your penis, says Sandra Hilton, PT, DPT, a doctor of physical therapy at Entropy Physiotherapy and Wellness in Chicago.

Once you feel how to contract and release your PC muscles, tighten and hold for a count of ten, then release. Practice in sets of ten. The beauty of this exercise, which will result in heightened ejaculatory control and help you last longer in bed? You can do it practically anywhere.

Practice edging.

Delaying your orgasm while masturbating can be one of the most effective ways to train yourself to last longer during sex. This is known as *edging*. Basically, you bring yourself right to the metaphorical "edge" of orgasm before stopping all sexual or masturbatory activity until you have your excitement under control. Then you start up again, repeating the process. After doing this about three or four times, you allow yourself to climax.

"Practicing this technique alone can help you teach your brain and body to better control your orgasm response and make [partnered] sex last longer," Brahmbhatt says. But it's also a fun thing you can do with your partner. *They* can edge you and see you squirm as they bring you to the brink of orgasm before stopping.

Try "the squeeze."

If you can feel your orgasm coming on, stop and squeeze right below the head of your penis. Apply firm pressure with your thumb and forefinger and focus the pressure on the urethra, the tube running along the underside of the penis, our chapter 3 sexpert Ian Kerner says. The squeeze technique can delay orgasm by pushing blood out of the penis, thereby repressing the ejaculatory response.

Masturbate beforehand.

Masturbating alone before a sexual encounter is a free and straightforward technique to help fight premature ejaculation. When you masturbate close to when you know you're going to have sex, you're essentially having sex a second time, which means it will take longer to climax. Of course, the issue with this is that you might not know when you're going to have sex, and you can't be on a date and run to the bathroom for a quick jerk before heading back to their place. You also need to time it well, because the last thing you want is not being able to perform at all.

Try numbing products.

Some sprays and anesthetic wipes contain numbing agents that make you last longer. Most work by simply spraying it (or rubbing the wipe) on your penis ten minutes before intercourse. Sex will still feel good; it just dulls the sensation so you can keep on pumping.

Wait longer for intercourse—or, hell, don't do it at all.

All too often, we think of sex as being penis-in-vagina or penis-in-anus. But that's such a limiting and, frankly, boring definition of sex. There are plenty of other sexual activities that'll both bring you pleasure and prolong the overall length of your hookup, including erotic massage, experimenting with kinks, or focusing entirely on stimulating your partner. (Oral sex, anyone?)

Keep going after you ejaculate.

All right, this isn't a tip to last longer, but it's crucial to reiterate: Sex does not have to be over just because you orgasmed. You can still make out, finger, suck, and go down on your partner until the cows come home. You can eat your partner out for so long that you actually get hard again and go a second time. You don't live in a porno. The camera of life doesn't stop rolling once you ejaculate.

WHAT'S UP WITH MY JUNK?

Does Size Matter?

Ah, the age-old question. We've all heard the phrase "it's not about the size of the boat; it's about the motion of the ocean." But is that just something guys with small dicks invented to make themselves feel better about their packages?

We're not going to lie to you. Yes, size does matter. If you have a three-inch penis when fully erect, your dating life is going to be more challenging than if you were packing a hefty seven inches. There will be certain people who will immediately dismiss you based on your penis size because they are size queens and have bought into societal messaging that having a big dick somehow equates to masculinity and sexual prowess. (Spoiler: It does not.)

But there's good news. While penis size *does* matter, it doesn't matter NEARLY as much as you think it does. There are also some tricks of the trade that can help you be a damn good lover without being hung like a horse.

But moving on, let's look at the facts: The average erect penis measures 5.16 inches, according to a 2015 scientific review published in *BJU International* that looked at the flaccid and erect penises of more than 15,500 men. In the review, 68 percent of men measured between 4.5 and 5.8 inches while erect.

BEST. SEX. EVER.

A lot of cis men, particularly straight cis men, have seen the erect penises only of porn stars, who are often packing eight, nine, or even ten inches. (There is a reason they are porn stars!) So if you've been watching porn your whole life, having seen the dicks of hundreds if not thousands of porn stars, you *likely* think your penis is tiny when it's perfectly average. After all, you're watching porn with guys whose dicks are *twice* the average size.

"I see a lot of men who are afraid that they have a small penis, but when I tell them to measure it, it turns out that it's perfectly average and sometimes even a little bigger than average," Brahmbhatt says.

So if this is you, check of the positions on pages 90–91 from Kerner.

Pro Tip: ➡ Use a Cock Ring for Stronger Erections

No matter what type of cock ring you use, they all work similarly: The ring traps blood inside the shaft of your penis, which helps you maintain an erection. Brahmbhatt prescribes special penis rings for patients who have venous leakage. "These men can get blood sent to the penis, but they have a 'leaky valve,' so they can't maintain an erection," he says. Cock rings solve this issue.

WHAT'S UP WITH MY JUNK?

But What Do I Do if I Actually Have a Small Penis?

Let's say you're packing three inches. Yes, there are procedures that you can do to enlarge your penis, but we don't recommend them because they are costly, potentially dangerous, and usually not super effective. For example, you *could* get a penile implant that can add 1.5 inches in length and 2.5 inches in girth, but it costs roughly $13,000 and you end up always being erect. Imagine trying to jog after that surgery. Or you could get fillers, which are cheaper, but they are temporary and impact the size of your penis only when flaccid, so not for sexual function.

Instead of trying to enhance your peen procedurally, let's focus on more practical and effective options.

Get damn good at going down on your partner.

If your partner has a vulva, become the best fucking pussy eater there is. Give them multiple orgasms without even sticking your dick inside of them. Then when you do eventually penetrate them with your dick, that will just be the icing on a very satisfying cake. If your partner has a penis, well, TBH, do some squats and become a big ol' power bottom. But also become the best dick sucker in all the land. Let go of the notion that sex *always* has to be P-in-V or P-in-B penetration, and that's just ridiculous.

Use penis sheaths.

Put these fantastic devices over your penis to increase your length or size. They come in various sizes, shapes, and textures and they're cheap to buy online. The best part is sex still feels great for you. It doesn't minimize your sensation.

Don't feel embarrassed or ashamed.

We know this is easier said than done, but you have nothing to feel bad about. And if you internalize that your worth is somehow connected to the size of your penis, you're going to be very unhappy. You won't be able to enjoy sex because you'll be so in your head. And remember, sex is just as much for you as it is for your partners. So relax and try the positions on page 88-89 from somatic psychologist and certified sex therapist Holly Richmond. You can still have fulfilling sex and find love.

Decentralize penetrative sex.

This won't be the last time you hear us say this: Sex isn't all about P-in-V or P-in-B penetration. FYI, many men aren't working with a "P" to begin with, and they're out there living their best sex lives. "There's this misconception that trans people are living in distress and can't have fulfilling sex lives, especially for straight, trans men like myself," says NYC-based therapist Stefan J. Simanovich, LCSW. "But that's just not true. I would argue we sometimes have more enriching sex lives because of needing to tap into different ways of having sex beyond penetrative sex."

Say What Now?

What's *Jelqing*?

Thanks to a few viral YouTube videos, there is an enthusiastic group of penis-owners out there who are huge proponents of jelqing, which purportedly increases the length and girth of your dick. Jelqing involves a series of exercises where you massage the base of your flaccid (or semi-chub) penis using your thumb and index finger. There hasn't been any legitimate research that supports that jelqing works, "and you can cause a lot of inflammation and potential scarring in your penis," Brahmbhatt says. "So it's not something that I recommend."

WHAT'S UP WITH MY JUNK?

THE BEST POSITIONS FOR...
PEOPLE WITH A SMALL PEEN

← **THE G-WHIZ**

With the receiver's legs over the giver's shoulders, this position allows for maximum depth. (Pro tip: Put a pillow under the receiver's lower back to achieve even more depth.) The giver can really go hard and deep with this one.

POLE POSITION →

While sitting on a bed, the receiver straddles one leg while facing away from the giver. Their hips will drop slightly more than in cowgirl, allowing for that extra penetration you want. The giver can use their hands to lift their partner's hips up and down.

BEST. SEX. EVER.

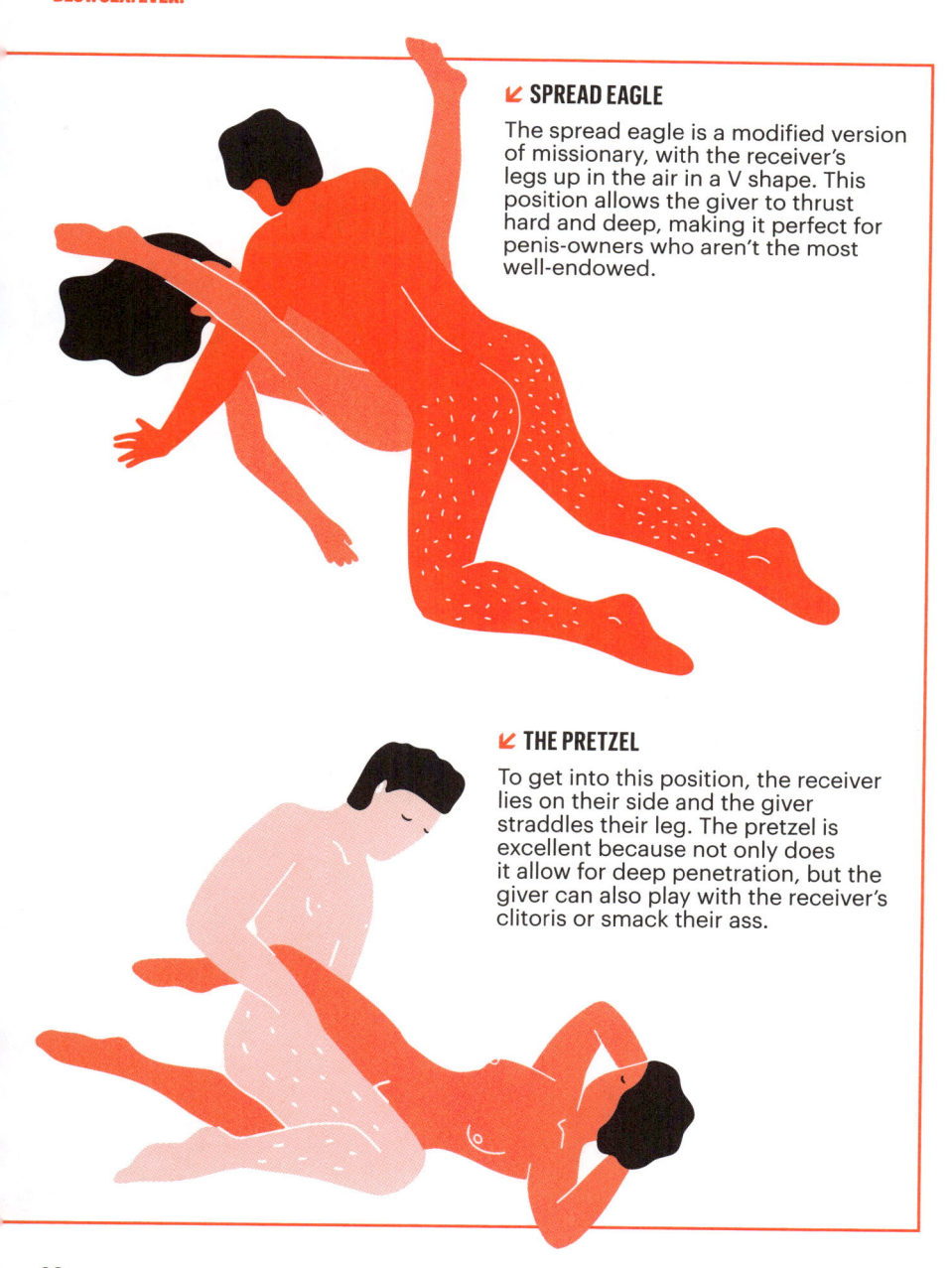

↙ SPREAD EAGLE

The spread eagle is a modified version of missionary, with the receiver's legs up in the air in a V shape. This position allows the giver to thrust hard and deep, making it perfect for penis-owners who aren't the most well-endowed.

↙ THE PRETZEL

To get into this position, the receiver lies on their side and the giver straddles their leg. The pretzel is excellent because not only does it allow for deep penetration, but the giver can also play with the receiver's clitoris or smack their ass.

WHAT'S UP WITH MY JUNK?

THE BEST POSITIONS FOR...
PEOPLE WITH A MEATY HOG

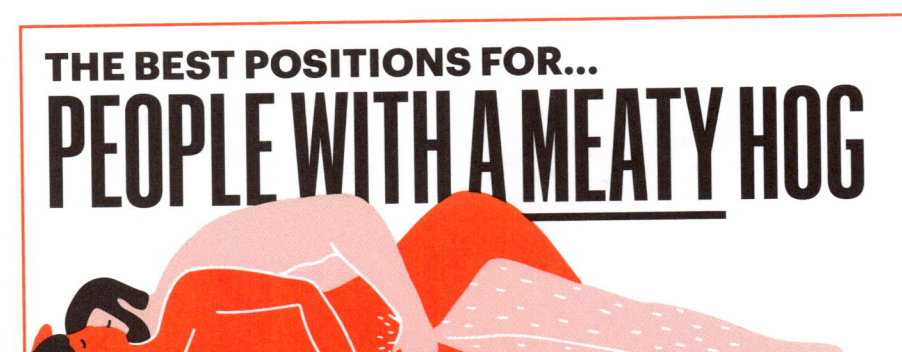

↑ OPEN-LEGGED SPOON

With the giver's legs pinned together by the weight of the receiver's leg, the receiver has control and good maneuvering ability, giving them the power to disengage with the giver's penis.

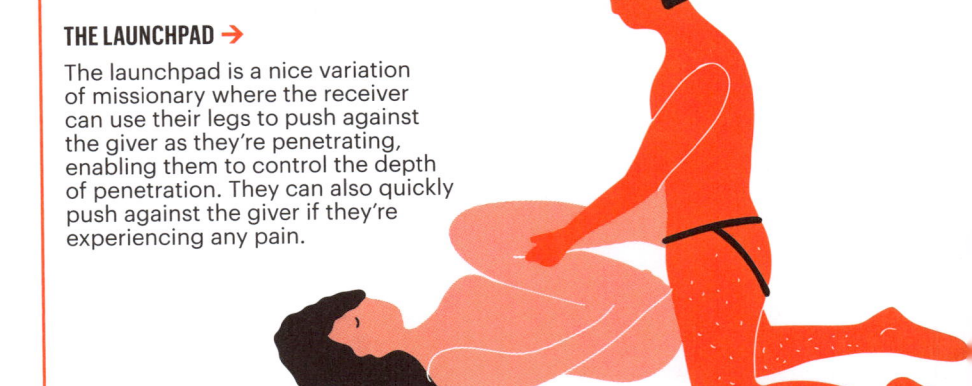

THE LAUNCHPAD →

The launchpad is a nice variation of missionary where the receiver can use their legs to push against the giver as they're penetrating, enabling them to control the depth of penetration. They can also quickly push against the giver if they're experiencing any pain.

BEST. SEX. EVER.

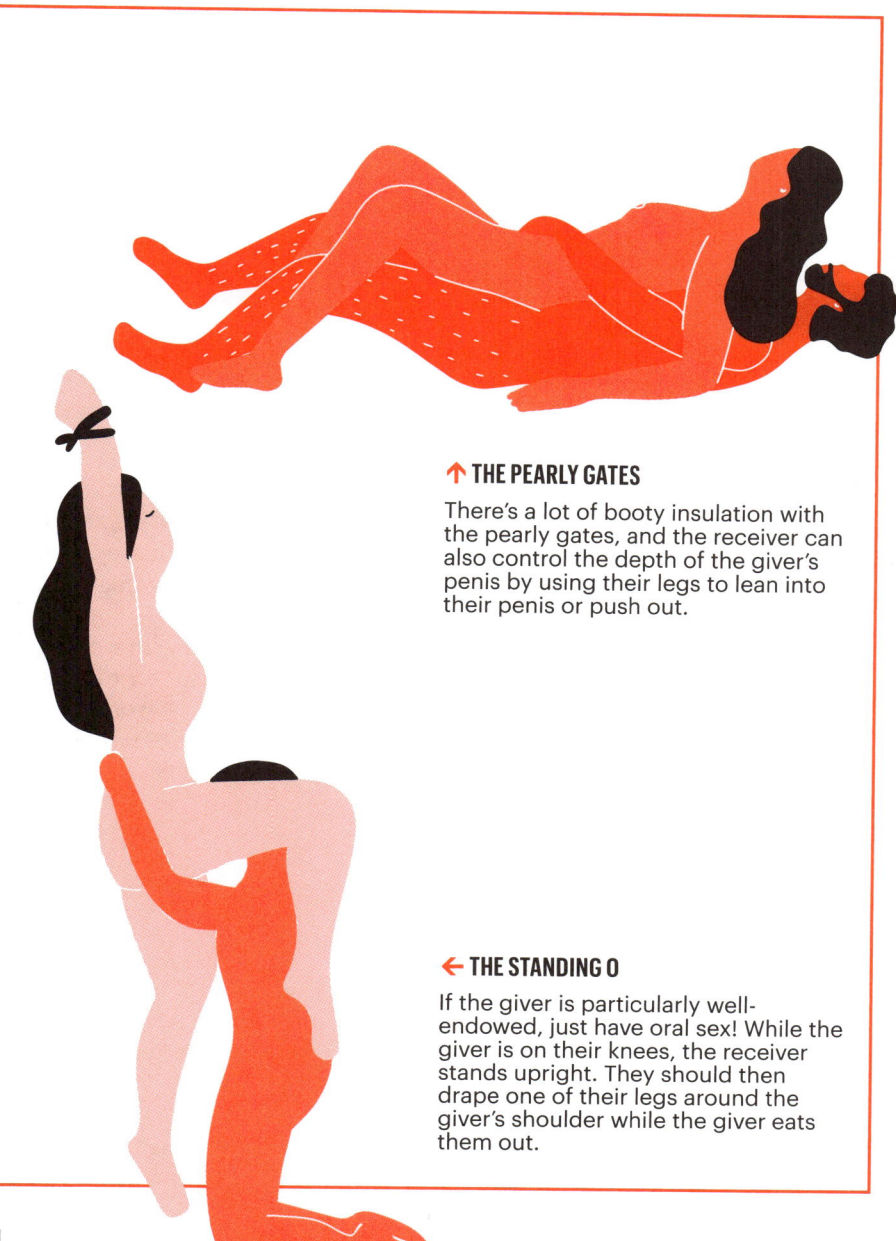

↑ THE PEARLY GATES

There's a lot of booty insulation with the pearly gates, and the receiver can also control the depth of the giver's penis by using their legs to lean into their penis or push out.

← THE STANDING O

If the giver is particularly well-endowed, just have oral sex! While the giver is on their knees, the receiver stands upright. They should then drape one of their legs around the giver's shoulder while the giver eats them out.

WHAT'S UP WITH MY JUNK?

SEXPLAIN IT

(a) ⟶ (b)

Dear Sexplain It,

I am a 43-year-old heterosexual Black man who has never been married and has no children. I also have a smaller-than-average penis. It's around five inches long and on the thinner side.

My penis size has caused very real problems in every relationship I've had. Many times, my partner couldn't even tell if I'd penetrated them or not. The therapist of one woman I dated encouraged her to tell me that my penis size (and sex) was an issue. It's really hurt my quality of life.

Not too long ago, I had a few experiences with women who were tighter/smaller, and sex felt great for the first time in years. Should I be patient and find a woman I can connect with in all the ways I would like or give up on the sexual satisfaction component of a relationship?

—Looking for the Right Fit

Dear Looking for the Right Fit,

I have news: Your penis isn't as small as you think it is.

The average erect penis is 5.16 inches long, and 90 percent of penis-owners fall within the range of 4 to 6.3 inches, notes a *BJU International* review. As for being on the "thinner side," the average girth (i.e., circumference) of a dick is 3.66 inches for a flaccid penis and 4.59 inches for an erect penis. I also want you to know there are plenty of women who will be able to feel you inside them: A report in *BJOG: An International Journal of Obstetrics and Gynaecology* found that the average depth of a vagina is about 3.77 inches. Although the vagina does expand when aroused, your five-inch peen's presence will certainly be known!

When I shared your question with sex and relationship expert Shamyra Howard, L.C.S.W., she suggested you may be feeling insecure about your totally average penis due to the "stereotype that Black men have the biggest cocks in the world." The idea is perpetuated in pop culture and porn—but it's not true. "When we're talking about penis size, there's no research that indicates that Black people have larger penises," says Howard.

Now, to answer your question: Please do NOT give up on the sexual satisfaction component of a relationship! You can and should find a woman you connect with emotionally *and* physically.

Let's talk about how to maximize your chances of success in the bedroom. The first step is beating the insecurity you have around your penis size. Whatever the root cause, your shame is probably affecting the way you approach sex. "You've had these issues regarding your penis size and performance before, so you think it's going to happen again," Howard says. "You're likely creating a self-fulfilling prophecy."

It's time to break that cycle and embrace the art of Big Dick Energy. There's a reason it's called Big Dick Energy (BDE) and not Actual Big Dick (ABD). Even if you don't have the world's biggest peen, people are attracted to a man who acts like he does. No matter how well you're endowed, women will be drawn to your confidence—

WHAT'S UP WITH MY JUNK?

your *swagger*—as long as you don't go overboard and enter into overcompensating-jerk territory.

Cultivating BDE isn't a panacea. There are certainly size queens who won't want to date you or fuck you because of your average-size dick, and you're never going to satisfy them. But the vast majority of women won't scoff at an average penis if you are confident in yourself and know how to use what you've got.

Next, I want you to shift your focus away from P-in-V penetration. "Sex is more about the physical, mental, emotional, and erotic connection shared between the people involved, and this is often done without penetration," Howard says.

Besides, most women can't orgasm from penetration alone. They also need direct clitoral stimulation—which is why you should learn how to get freaking great at fingering and oral sex.

And take your time. So many guys do this 50-seconds-of-fingering-before-sticking-your-dick-in business. If that happens to be you, cut that shit out.

I also want to encourage you to start bringing sex toys into the bedroom. I don't care how big your dick is: It still can't vibrate. It still can't suction a clitoris while achieving maximum depth and G-spot penetration. Your dick isn't a magic wand, but do you know what is? The actual Magic Wand.

But above all else, just remember: It's all about that BDE, not ABD.

BEST. SEX. EVER.

5

BUTT STUFF

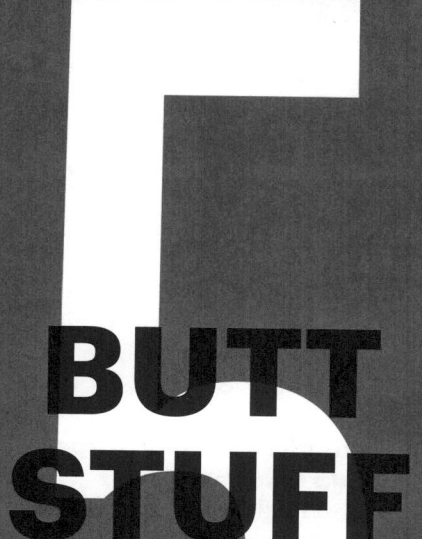

YOUR SEXPERT

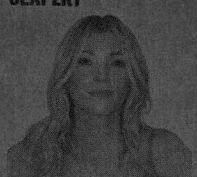

Certified sex educator **Alicia Sinclair** is the founder and CEO of b-Vibe, a line of innovative vibrating anal toys known for its rimming and weighted butt plugs.

> Most guys love a good ass, but when it comes to getting our own booties involved during sex, some of us are reluctant. Here you'll learn the ins and outs (pun intended) of anal play—both receiving and giving.

CHAPTER

BUTT STUFF

How Do I Get Over the Stigma of Anal Play?

Let's start off with a simple question. Why does butt stuff feel pleasurable?
SINCLAIR: For the same reason that "front stuff" feels pleasurable! There are tons of nerve endings in the anal canal. At the entry of the bum, there's also the anal sphincter, which has 4,000 nerve endings, which is the same number of nerve endings as the head of the penis and about half as many as the clitoris.

How does anal stimulation differ in sensation depending on whether you have a penis or vulva?
If you have a penis, you most likely have a prostate, a walnut-size gland located below the bladder and in front of the rectum. It is located about two inches inside your anus and faces up toward your belly button. If you were to lie down flat on your back, your partner could stimulate it by making a "come hither" motion with their fingers. If you have a vulva, the pressure inside the anal canal shares space with the vaginal canal. So it's possible to stimulate clusters of the internal clitoris, including the G-spot and the deeper A-spot [anterior fornix erogenous zone], through anal stimulation.

Anal play isn't pleasurable only because of anatomy. There are also psychological factors that contribute to why so many folks get turned on by butt stuff. What are they?
They say the mind is the biggest sex organ, and as somebody who identifies as a woman, I would say that it sometimes feels good to be "slutty." There's something that is very daring and goes against that "good girl" concept of how you're supposed to have sex when you're having anal.

You're having this "raunchy" sex—and that, mentally, can be a huge turn-on.

And say if you're a guy? What do men get out of having something or someone inside their rear ends?
It creates a shift in power dynamics. Men are typically dominant. But when penetrated, it provides an opportunity to be more submissive, and many men, along with women, love the role reversal. (Women like being able to feel more dominant when pegging or simply just inserting fingers inside a man!) It brings a totally unique experience physically, emotionally, and even spiritually.

It's clear that anal play has physical and psychological benefits for men, so why are so many guys—especially straight guys—afraid to try it?
When I teach anal trainings, inevitably one woman says, "My boyfriend really likes receiving anal sex. Does that make him gay?" This is a really common misconception. There's this false idea that liking anal play has something to do with sexual orientation. There's also so much social conditioning around how a man is supposed to act and what equals "manhood" and "strength." Men, and women too, have been taught that if a man likes anal on himself or enjoys being submissive, then he's not a "real man." But the truth is, being submissive or receptive has nothing to do with your manhood.

How can those guys get over the stigma and actually give it a try?
Guys have to remember this: The sensations and experiences that feel good have nothing to do with your sexual orientation or gender. There's nothing inherently feminine about receiving anal stimulation and penetration. You get to decide what anal play means to you and how you feel about it. And when you can let go of the idea that a sexual act has to be done by a specific gender, you'll discover some amazing opportunities.

BUTT STUFF

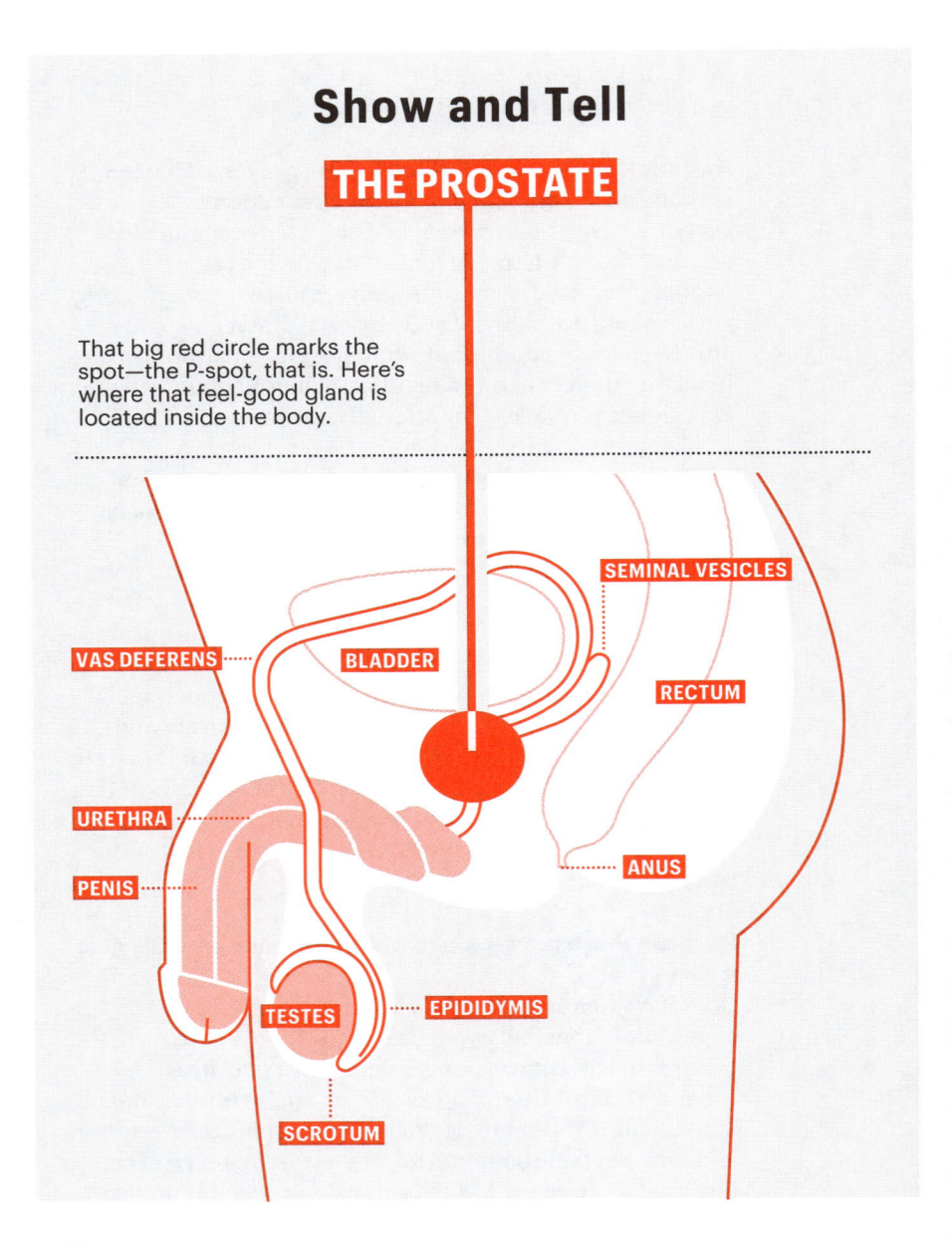

Show and Tell

THE PROSTATE

That big red circle marks the spot—the P-spot, that is. Here's where that feel-good gland is located inside the body.

- VAS DEFERENS
- BLADDER
- SEMINAL VESICLES
- RECTUM
- URETHRA
- PENIS
- ANUS
- TESTES
- EPIDIDYMIS
- SCROTUM

BEST. SEX. EVER.

Why Do People Love Anal Sex So Damn Much?

We wouldn't encourage you to explore anal sex if it weren't enjoyable. It takes a lot of effort to prepare for anal sex, so if the gain were minimal, we wouldn't put you through the rigmarole.

But anal sex *is* that good. Don't just take our word for it. We reached out to numerous gay, straight, and bisexual men to learn what they love about giving and receiving anal sex, both physically and psychologically. Flip to the next page to read their responses about why the love topping or bottoming.

Pro Tip: ➡ Did You Use Enough LUBE?!

Repeat after us: Spit does not count as lube. The anus, unlike the vagina, is not self-lubricating, meaning that you should apply a lot of lube often. While booty aficionados prefer silicone-based lube for anal sex because it is thicker and lasts longer, you can't use silicone-based lube with silicone toys. (It'll erode and eventually destroy the toy.) So you want to use a water-based lube when going to town with a silicone butt plug, anal beads, or a dildo.

BUTT STUFF

CONFESSIONS

"Why I Love Topping…"

"Like most guys, I enjoy a nice butt. Something about a plump, round ass really turns me on and drives me crazy. And a tight hole feels fucking incredible. And I love being able to dominate a big, masculine, manly man. That's definitely not how I look, so I feel like I'm fucking with the male patriarchy and toxic masculinity with each muscle bottom I fuck." —**Brandon, 27**

"The first time I pegged my boyfriend went fabulously, so much so that I actually came while fucking him! What I loved was how in control I felt, how sexy I knew I looked, and, when I wanted to, how intimate I could make the situation. I was turning myself on!" —**Kellan, 20**

"I enjoy how the inside of an anus feels thrusting against my hard penis. It doesn't get better than when your eyes roll to the back of your head while ejaculating into a tight asshole. I also love the feeling of being in complete sexual control of someone who wants me deep inside of them." —**Michael, 35**

"I love how it can be deeply intimate. The male partners I have pegged have all expressed a deeper appreciation for the art and skill set of receiving, and in that moment, I feel more seen, understood, and appreciated. It's easy to think—especially in straight culture—that bottoming is easy, but once you have a dick in your ass, you learn real quickly that it can require lots of emotional and physical release. In this way, I feel safer and more understood by men who have bottomed." —**Crystal, 41**

BEST. SEX. EVER.

CONFESSIONS

"Why I Love Bottoming…"

"I love the orgasms! I find it hard to have multiple orgasms when I top, but when I bottom properly, it feels like the world moves through me every time I cum, and I'm immediately ready to go again. It's a weird sensation physically. On the one hand, there's the need for relaxing and releasing, but on the other, there's a lot of contracting. And where topping activates my mind in a way, bottoming sort of quiets it. I get to focus on nothing but pleasure and release." **—Grey, 30**

"I love a whole lot [about getting pegged]. For one, better orgasms. I would say the difference between a 'normal' intercourse orgasm and the ones from pegging is threefold. I can get a full-body orgasm and occasionally multiple ones. Second, it feels nice to be filled. I know that women often report this and some of my gay mates do too, so I guess that is the right expression. Third, it's much more emotionally intense. And lastly, it's simply nice not to be the active partner for a change. Ninety percent of my sex is still pretty 'classic,' where I control the action, so variety is definitely a factor here." **—John, 35**

"The physical and psychological pleasures of bottoming kinda blend for me. I've rarely had as intense a sexual experience as bottoming. When it's good, it's otherworldly. As a biggish (six-foot-two) guy who had mainly slept with women, having another guy dominate me physically is overwhelming. It taught me so much about power and trust and safety and masculinity. It skirts along that line between pain and pleasure—control and release." **—Joe, 31**

BUTT STUFF

What About Poop?

There's always one big question newbies have when it comes to anal sex: What about poop? Valid question! After all, expelling feces is the primary purpose of the anus and rectum.

But here's a little anatomy lesson: The rectum does not store feces. Feces transfer from the intestines and are pushed out through your rectum and then anus. This is important to remember because a lot of folks have this idea that your poop is just sitting right inside your butthole. Untrue! You're not going to "hit" a piece of poop if you start poking around up there.

Luckily, through diet, fiber supplements, cleaning out (i.e., douching), and familiarizing yourself with your own body, you can drastically decrease the likelihood of having any brown specks during your sexual encounter.

Diet

Bottoming isn't just an activity; it's a lifestyle. It's something that people prepare for over the course of their day (or even weeks). If a guy is bottoming daily or almost daily, you'll notice that they have a very strict diet. That's because they want to be ready to take a penis or dildo in their rear end at any moment. (God bless!)

The key to maintaining a healthy bowel system—which decreases the likelihood of having a poopy sexual encounter—is fiber intake. Fiber keeps your bowel system regular and moving, which is what you want! Luckily, foods high in fiber are predominantly healthy, so you're killing two birds with one stone. Most fruits and vegetables have a lot of fiber, including raspberries, pears, apples, bananas, carrots, cauliflower, and broccoli. You can also eat whole-grain foods, potatoes, and nuts.

Now, if having a fiber-rich diet sounds exhausting or limiting, you can also take Metamucil. (Note: When you're eating fiber-rich foods or taking Metamucil, you must drink plenty of water; otherwise, you may feel constipated or bloated.)

As for what not to eat? Typically, you want to avoid any greasy, fried, fatty, creamy, heavy, or spicy foods that can upset your stomach. You also may want to steer clear of excessive alcohol and caffeine because they can cause your bowels to move a little *too* quickly, if you catch our drift.

Prepping

Some guys can get away with just eating properly and never have to clean out their rectum. As for the rest of us? We need to wash!

"Anal preparation is very personal, and folks have different opinions on it," Sinclair says. That said, there are two main ways you can clean out your ass: douching with a little bulb, where you squeeze clean water into your behind, and using a hose that you can connect to your showerhead and insert into your butt (often referred to as a shower enema).

Let's start with a douche bulb. You want to fill up the bulb with clean water (from the tap is fine). Don't use hot water or you will burn your insides; use tepid or cold water! Then you insert the bulb nozzle into your rear end. You can lube up the nozzle too, which helps it glide inside of you. From there, lightly pump water into your asshole by squeezing the bulb.

Remember, you're trying to clean out your rectum. (Need a quick anatomy lesson? Turn to page 98.) If you pump too quickly (or use too much water), you'll accidentally squirt too far up in your butt, past your rectum and into your lower intestines. This will cause an avalanche of poop to come out of your behind, and you'll have to keep on cleaning. The douching process that was supposed

BUTT STUFF

to take only five to ten minutes will now take between 45 minutes and an hour and a half.

All right, once you've squirted the water into your rectum, go ahead and sit over a toilet and expel it. Don't strain! Your rectum will feel full, so your body will naturally want to release the water. You want to repeat this until the water runs clear (i.e., there's no fecal matter coming out and the water isn't brown). Really, when douching, you don't want to use more than two full bulbs. (Most bulbs are between seven and ten ounces; don't get any that are bigger than that!) Over-douching is very much a thing—an epidemic!—and you can damage the inner lining in your butt, which puts you at a higher risk for sexually transmitted infections.

Now on to shower hoses. Shower hoses do purposely clean out your lower intestines, making you squeaky clean, but this makes the cleaning process much longer.

Just like with a douche, you insert the hose into your rear end. Then you turn on the shower and it shoots water into you. It can be difficult to control pressure with a shower hose, so please be careful. Then, instead of expelling over the toilet, you simply expel over the shower drain.

Hoses are definitely for more advanced bottoms; the average man doesn't need to use one. Hoses are ideal if you plan on having anal sex for a long period of time or if you plan on taking a particularly long penis or dildo. If you're just putting a butt plug inside of yourself or your partner is going to put in only a couple of fingers, then this level of cleanliness is unnecessary.

Whether you douche or use a hose, "give yourself about an hour before your anal play experience because sometimes water gets trapped in the folds of your squiggly little anal canal, so you can have a little extra water come out," Sinclair says.

What if I'm Still Not Clean?

Sometimes you can eat perfectly and douche meticulously, but you still make a little mess. Shit happens—literally! There's no reason to apologize profusely, and you definitely don't need to feel any shame or embarrassment. After all, it's your goddamn butthole. Your partner knew what they were getting into. Like, what? They're going to be surprised that some poop comes out of your butt? That's where shit comes from, buddy!

(Also, it's worth noting that there will likely be a little bit of poop flakes. It's not like you're going to take a huge dump on your partner! To be honest, the smell is worse than what little specks of feces actually come out.)

Oh, and if they in any way shame you for not being clean, just know that they're the asshole here, not your asshole.

"If something [poop-related] happens, I think it's best to have a backup plan or emergency plan," Sinclair says. "That can be as simple as laying down a dark towel before sex, so if something happens, you can just fold the towel and throw it in the dirty clothes." Then you and your partner can go quickly shower and rinse yourselves off. "Once rinsed, you keep the sex going by moving on to another type of play that doesn't involve anal," she says.

BUTT STUFF

How Do I Warm Up That Bootyhole?

Just like how you walk before you run, you insert fingers before inserting anything else of substantial size up your or your partner's bum. Slow and steady wins the race here. There is absolutely no reason to rush, and it's not a competition either. Take only what you can take. This isn't a "push through the pain" situation. This is an "if it hurts, stop, slow down, and go back to something tinier" situation.

How Do I Prepare to Finger Someone's Anus?

If you're fingering someone, the first thing you need to do before even getting close to your partner's anus is cut your fingernails (and file them down), says Evan Goldstein, D.O., founder and CEO of the anal surgery practice, Bespoke Surgical. When you have long nails or jagged edges, you can accidentally scratch your partner's rectum, which is as painful as it sounds! Wash your hands too! Let's not add any more bacteria to what's already up in there.

What Are the Best Positions for Anal Fingering?

There are three traditional positions for anal fingering. The first is when the receiver is on their stomach in a starfish. The second is in a doggy-style position, and the third is when they're on their back with their legs up in the air. "I recommend positions like these that give you or your partner a clear view of the hole," Goldstein says. "If you can see it—and I mean all of it—then you have a better chance of understanding the angles and anatomy to make the experience most pleasurable."

Should I Be Using Lube?

Lube is not optional when it comes to anal fingering. It's mandatory! You specifically want "long-lasting lubes like silicone-based or oil-based lubes," says sex and pleasure educator Luna Matatas. And make sure to apply lube both on your finger(s) and directly on and around the anus. Reapply it generously and frequently.

How Do I Start?

The most common issue that can happen with anal fingering is tearing, otherwise known as anal fissures," Goldstein says. This can happen when you thrust or insert too much too quickly. That's why, before even starting with a finger, you should massage the external anus "as if you're petting the butthole," Matatas says. This helps the anal muscles relax.

What's the Tempo for Digital Penetration?

After you've teased their hole with external play, you can *slowly* insert a finger before eventually working your way up to two or more (if you ever reach that point). Take your time. Again, there's no rush to put in more (and you may just want to stick to one little pinky finger if it's your or your partner's first time). When in doubt, ask your partner if they want more.

Should I Focus on the "In and Out"?

"The anus doesn't only get pleasure from depth, so try moving your finger so you're massaging the sides of the anus in a horizontal motion," Matatas says. And remember, the prostate is two to three inches inside your anus. That's the money maker and what feels really good when stimulated. So you want to focus on that part of the region when fingering or getting fingered.

BUTT STUFF

THE BUYER$ GUIDE TO...
ANAL TOYS

BUTT PLUGS are teardrop-shaped toys, typically made of silicone, metal, or glass. Some vibrate; others have rotating beads at the base of the toy to simulate rimming. Pop a butt plug in your rear end and let it rest there for a satisfying feeling of fullness.

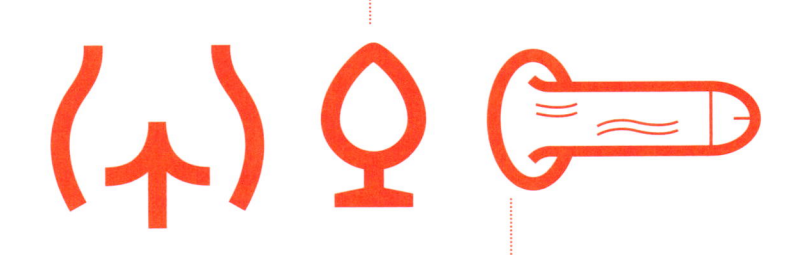

There is a wide range of anal sex toys depending on what you're hoping to get out of the experience and which sensations you find most pleasurable. Remember: Don't put a toy (or anything else!) in your butt unless it has a flared base.

DILDOS is an all-encompassing word for sex toys designed for penetration. They come in many shapes and sizes: Some look like a realistic penis, whereas others are more abstract. Dildos are great for anal aficionados looking for bigger and better things. You can ride a dildo or thrust it in and out of yourself while you're on your back. You can even get dildos that suction to a wall if you want to replicate doggy style on your own.

BEST. SEX. EVER.

ANAL BEADS look kind of like rosary beads, except chunkier, and instead of praying with them, you put them in your butt. While you absolutely can use anal beads for solo play, they're fun to use with a partner since they're more interactive. "Anal beads are designed to stimulate the anal sphincter through movement," Sinclair explains. When pulled out, each sphere delivers a quick burst of intense sensation. Part of the fun of anal beads is seeing how many of them you can take, but it's also relinquishing control to your partner. They can pop each one out and watch you shake with pleasure.

PROSTATE MASSAGERS are toys that are curved to target your prostate and deliver earth-shattering, toe-curling, full-body orgasms. (Typically, they vibrate too!) There are two main types of prostate massagers: ones with perineum stimulation and ones without. (The *perineum*, aka the taint or grundle, is that strip of skin between your testicles/vulva and your anus.) Those with perineum stimulation are typically V- or C-shaped; not only does the extra arm provide added pressure to the often ignored erogenous zone, but it also helps keep the prostate massager in place.

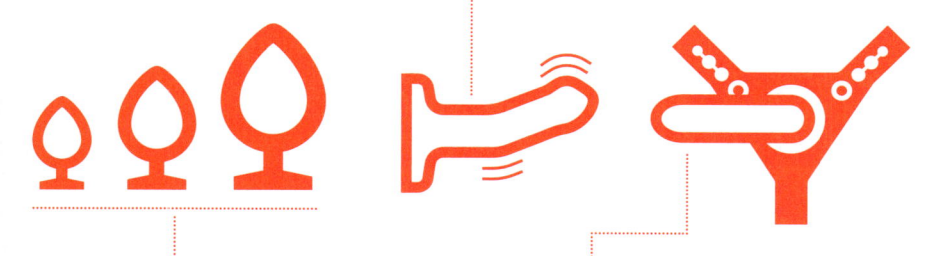

ANAL TRAINING KITS are perfect if you are new to anal play and want to work your way up to taking a penis or dildo. These kits include a pack of butt plugs in different sizes. Start with the smallest one and wear it until you're used to the sensation. When it's fitting comfortably to the point where you can easily insert and remove it, move up to the next plug.

PEGGING EQUIPMENT—i.e., a harness and dildo—allows someone who doesn't have a penis to penetrate their partner. Pegging is a whole experience. It's not just about the physical sensation; it's also intimate, vulnerable, and great for tapping into your more submissive side if you're the one on the receiving end.

BUTT STUFF

How Do I Eat the Booty Like Groceries?

The first time you learned about anilingus—also known as rimming, tossing salad, ass eating, peach munching, eating the booty like groceries—you probably thought to yourself, *Wait, people seriously do this? What the flying fuck?!* Yes, all kinds of couples enjoy eating some delicious booty.

"You definitely want to make sure that you have prepared before rimming," Sinclair says. "It's going to be a pretty intimate experience."

It may sound a little gross or unsanitary, but douching and thoroughly washing the external anus with soap and water significantly decreases the likelihood of passing any icky bacteria. It also gets rid of any unappealing taste that may linger. (Turn to page 103 to learn how to douche.)

How Do I Start Eating Ass?

"A lot of people have this perception that they don't need to do any foreplay with rimming, but just like with every other type of sexual experience, you want to warm up," Sinclair says. That means you don't quickly pull your partner's ass cheeks apart and ram your tongue in and out of their anus as fast as you can.

"Start by teasing the anus," she says. "Make circles with your tongue, lick it like ice cream, and play with the entire booty. Really get your hands on it. Spank it. Shake it!" Once they're warmed up and begging for more, that's when you can really get all up in there using a wide variety of techniques.

What Are the Best Techniques for Eating Ass?

There's more to rimming than spreading those cheeks and feasting. I mean, you could do that, and honestly, you both might enjoy it, but you do have other options if you want to get creative. (Thank you Matatas for providing us with these tips!)

Flatten the top of your tongue against their anus.
This creates a larger surface area for your tongue, so your partner gets more wetness and pressure from every lick.

Use more than your tongue.
Your tongue will get tired quicker than you think. That's why it's great to use other parts of your face like your nose and chin, which apply different types of pressure to your partner's anus.

Give pleasure to surrounding anal areas.
Sure, the anus is the most sensitive, but you still have a full booty to play with. Lick the butt crack. Shake those cheeks. You can even use a sex toy to stimulate your partner's genitals and perineum.

Try a position where the receiver has control.
Try something like face-sitting, which gives more power to the receiver—they can move their butt to control where their anus lands on your tongue and chin.

BUTT STUFF

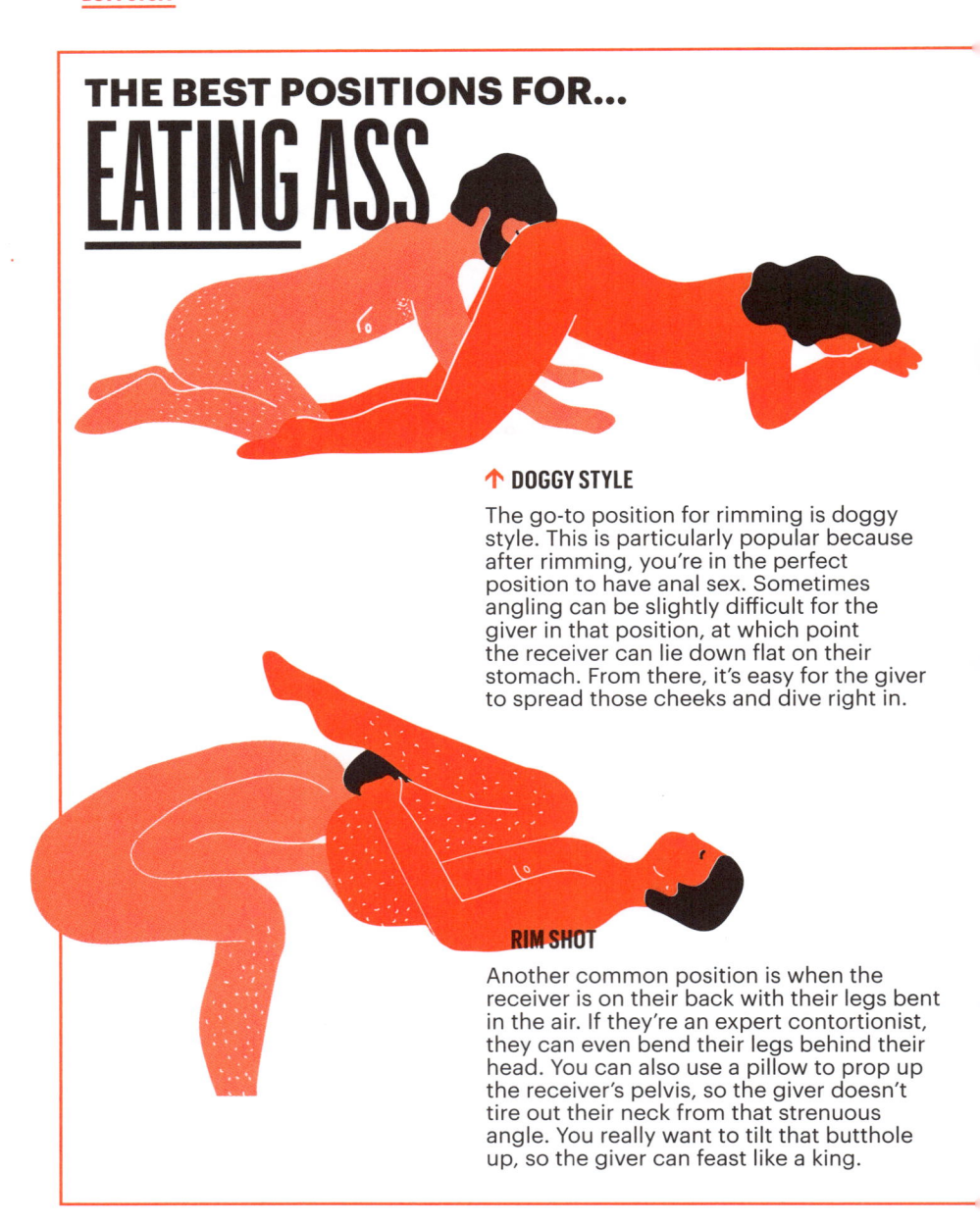

THE BEST POSITIONS FOR...
EATING ASS

↑ DOGGY STYLE

The go-to position for rimming is doggy style. This is particularly popular because after rimming, you're in the perfect position to have anal sex. Sometimes angling can be slightly difficult for the giver in that position, at which point the receiver can lie down flat on their stomach. From there, it's easy for the giver to spread those cheeks and dive right in.

RIM SHOT

Another common position is when the receiver is on their back with their legs bent in the air. If they're an expert contortionist, they can even bend their legs behind their head. You can also use a pillow to prop up the receiver's pelvis, so the giver doesn't tire out their neck from that strenuous angle. You really want to tilt that butthole up, so the giver can feast like a king.

BEST. SEX. EVER.

FACE-SITTING →

You need to be a little careful with this one. The receiver can't put *all* of their weight on their partner's face—that's just painful. It's helpful for the person being rimmed to use a bed or a wall to help balance their weight off their knees and thighs and control how much ass they put on their partner's face.

↙ REVERSE FACE-SIT

Here, the receiver sits on the giver's face but faces away from them. This position is popular among guys who love to be completely smothered by booty, even to the point where they can't breathe. It combines a big-booty fetish with breath play (i.e., asphyxiation).

ANILINGUS 69 ↘

While one person's eating some booty, the other person can perform oral at the same time. It's a win-win!

BUTT STUFF

THE BEST POSITIONS FOR...
ANAL SEX THAT AREN'T DOGGY STYLE

↙ THE ZODIAC

While seated in a chair (or at the end of the bed), the receiving partner straddles the giver, facing toward them, and wraps their legs around them. This is an intimate position that allows for making out, caressing, and holding. All too often, we think of "taking them from behind" for anal sex, but face-to-face positions can be very romantic.

THE CAPTAIN →

Oh captain, my captain! The receiver lies on their back and holds their legs up straight in a V shape. This grants the top full access to their booty, and they can really pound hard in this one, if that's your vibe.

BEST. SEX. EVER.

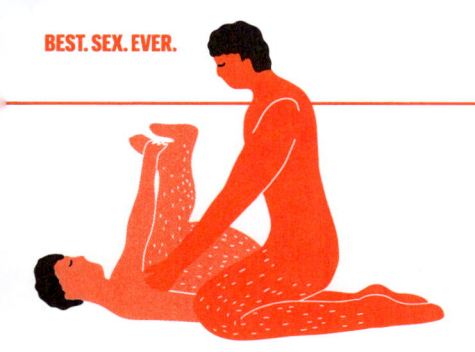

HAPPY BABY POSE ↑

The receiver lies on their back and throws their bent legs up into the air. Their legs should be slightly past shoulder width apart, and for this pose to really work, they need to grip the soles of their feet with their hands. This allows for deeper penetration, and if the receiver is a vulva-owner, it's also an ideal position for engaging their clit.

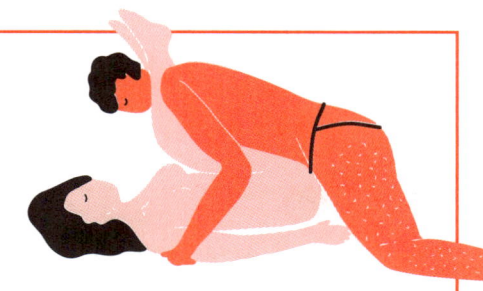

LEGS ON SHOULDERS ↑

While the receiver is on their back, they drape their legs over the top's shoulders. The angle of their body should be roughly 90 degrees. The legs-on-shoulders position should be considered a staple, as it allows for deep anal penetration.

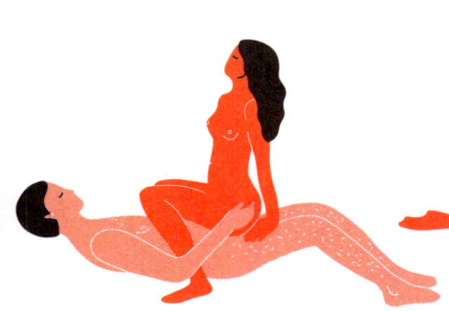

SQUATTING COWGIRL ↑

It's similar to traditional cowgirl, where the giver's on their back and the receiver straddles them. Only instead of the receiver having their knees beside the giver, they have their soles planted on the bed in a squatting position. With this position, the giver can grab them by the butt and thrust deeply. Even though their partner's on top, the giver's still in control of the speed and motion.

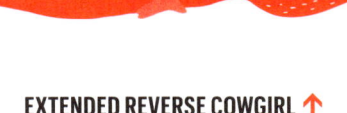

EXTENDED REVERSE COWGIRL ↑

The receiver hops on top of the giver, facing the opposite direction, like it's reverse cowgirl. Then they lean back, planting the palms of their hands by the sides of their partner's shoulders or face, depending on their height. Typical reverse cowgirl is tough to pull off in anal because of the angle. Extended reverse cowgirl solves this problem.

BUTT STUFF

SEXPLAIN IT

Dear Sexplain It,

Zach, I've been reading all your articles on anal/prostate play for men and I finally decided to try it out alone. It felt incredible. So then I started doing anal play stuff with my girlfriend. I was surprised how into it she was too. Now we use anal beads, butt plugs, etc. all the time.

The issue is, now I can't orgasm without something inside me. This is for both masturbation and sex. It just doesn't feel as good. I guess my body is used to this heightened sensation, so I need it to finish. It's annoying, because you have to prep for anal sex, and I don't want to/can't every time. I'm not trying to douche for 45 minutes just because I want to masturbate for five.

How do I get back to the point where I can orgasm without something inside me?

—Obsessed With Anal

Dear Obsessed With Anal,

I'm tearing up from joy. My bottom agenda has finally come to fruition. More men are exploring the depths of our rear end, and we're embracing the mind-blowing ecstasy that comes with anal stimulation. In your case, a little too much ecstasy, as you're struggling to orgasm without something in your ass.

This makes perfect sense. You've tapped into a treasure trove of sexual pleasure that takes your orgasms to new heights. Your body is now accustomed to this extreme pleasure—it has a new threshold for physiological arousal—so it can't orgasm without reaching this new bar.

I think there's a possibility this will autocorrect on its own in time. Think about how it felt to discover (non-booty) masturbation for the first time. You probably wanted to jack off all day, every day! Eventually—I assume—you learned to live without masturbating 24/7. I think the same will hold true for your anal obsession.

You're still relatively new to anal play. I remember when I first discovered anal play, I couldn't get enough of it. I always wanted something in my ass while having sex. My girlfriend at the time joked about opening Pandora's box by introducing me to anal. Ultimately, my fixation faded. Nothing happened, *per se*. There were just a few times when I couldn't do anal because of my bowels, so we had regular sex and I enjoyed it (almost) as much. Now I can easily have euphoric sex without something inside my butt. Do I still love having something in my booty? Of course! But I consider it a little treat as opposed to a must-have.

All right, as for weaning you off anal play, I asked your question to booty expert Luna Matatas. First and foremost, she recommends taking a break from insertable butt stuff. It can take anywhere between a few days and a few weeks to recalibrate, depending on how much masturbatory or partnered sex you've been having. Also: "Taking a break from orgasming altogether for a few days can jump-start this process of heightening arousal," she adds. So let's not have sex or jerk off for a few days, then return to non-booty sex stuff.

BUTT STUFF

Once you're able to orgasm without something in your butt, just do that for a few weeks. Then you can start reintegrating anal play back into your sexual repertoire. When you eventually do, take it slow. If you dive headfirst into having sex with a giant butt plug in and do so every day for two weeks, you'll likely end up back at square one.

However…I also kinda think you should lean into being a big ol' bottom?

Your issue with anal play is the prep it takes to bottom. Here's some good news: You are drastically overprepping. You don't need to douche for 45 minutes if you're taking two fingers or a three-inch vibrating butt plug in your rear end. You need to douche that thoroughly if you're preparing for some eight-inch dick (or dildo). If you're taking something on the smaller side, you can actually douche with one bulb, two tops. (This will take all of five minutes.)

Taking fiber pills can also make the douching process much quicker—everything flows more smoothly down there. (You'll come to learn you may not even need to douche at all once you start taking fiber pills.)

So keep getting your prostate involved through both external and internal stimulation. Enjoy those earth-shattering orgasms that come with something in or around your anus. Be the big ol' bottom God wanted you to be. Life's too short not to shove things up your ass.

BEST. SEX. EVER.

YOUR SEXPERT

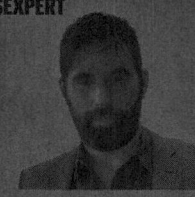

Justin Lehmiller, Ph.D., is a *Men's Health* advisory panel member, a research fellow at the Kinsey Institute, and the author of *Tell Me What You Want*.

KINKS AND FETISHES

As the saying goes, "We all have our kinks." But exactly how common are kinks, where do they come from, and why are they considered "deviant"?

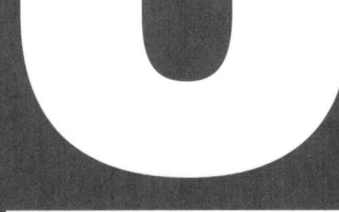

CHAPTER 6

KINKS AND FETISHES

Are My Kinks Normal?

People tend to use *kinks* and *fetishes* interchangeably, but isn't there actually a difference?
LEHMILLER: Yes, *kink* is an umbrella term that refers to any type of sexual interest that falls outside of the mainstream. It can be any number of things, including BDSM [bondage and discipline, dominance and submission, sadism, and masochism], choking, and role play. A *fetish* tends to refer more to a specific object or non-genital body part that often is essential for sexual arousal.

There's more on kinks later in the chapter, but what are some common fetishes?
The most common fetish objects tend to surround the feet, legs, or genitals—so underwear, bras, panties, lingerie, boots, and shoes. But I've heard about fetishes for dirt, cars, and the radio. There are also several fetishes involving medical tools and doctor settings, so a speculum or lab coat. I've even heard of folks with fetishes for pacemakers, which involves a dominant-submissive component. Basically, one person has control over the other person's heartbeat.

That's definitely a life-changing fetish. Where might a fetish like that come from?

There are a lot of different things that can draw someone to a kink or fetish. The most common explanation is that kinks and fetishes are learned early on in life—a certain object or activity was paired with sexual arousal and there was a powerful orgasm. This created an association that made them want to repeat that experience. But that's not to say that kinks and fetishes can be learned only during adolescence. Some people develop them later in life, like when an older adult with a chronic illness turns to BDSM to cope with pain. It can also be something that a partner introduces you to and then you find it pleasurable.

In my own research, I've found links between certain personality traits and kinks and fetishes. When you consider that personality traits are at least partially heritable, that would suggest a genetic contribution that predisposes individuals to develop certain kinks and fetishes.

So if you have a kink to call someone "Daddy," that may have come from your actual daddy? Oh, boy. Well, instead of unpacking that, please explain why there is such a stigma toward BDSM and kinks.

One reason is that our ideas about sex and sexual morality have a long religious history behind them. In many of the dominant religions, the definition of what is "normal" and moral when it comes to sex is very limited and often refers only to penile-vaginal intercourse in the context of a heterosexual, monogamous marriage and procreation. Since we're taught this from a young age, it's very easy to feel shame or weird or that something is wrong with us for having, really, *any* turn-on.

But another part of this has to do with how the mental health community has treated sexual interests throughout history. Historically, sadomasochism was considered to be a deviant sexual interest. Doctors thought that only somebody who has something really wrong with them would be turned on by BDSM. In fact, it wasn't that long ago that sadism and masochism were listed as disorders in the *DSM* [*Diagnostic and Statistical Manual of Mental Disorders*], which is the psychiatry bible. It's only been in the past decade that medical professionals have changed how they talk about kinks.

So now in the *DSM-5*, they have "sexual sadism disorder" and "sexual masochism disorder" rather than just "sadism" and "masochism." This updated terminology refers only to cases where somebody's sexual interest is causing distress and problems in their life because it's nonconsensual or creating some other type of problem. Increasingly, psychologists and psychiatrists make a distinction between having an unusual sexual interest and having a sexual disorder. That's been a really important shift in the field, but I don't think that the public is even aware of these changes.

It seems like this stigma is so deeply rooted in all of us. How do we get over any internalized shame we have around our kinky sexual desires?
Part of it is expanding your definition of what "normal" sex is and realizing how common these sexual interests are. When you start to understand how common some of these sexual interests are, it can help lead to self-acceptance. And self-acceptance is the first step to get over any shame you may feel regarding your kinky desires.

Only then, after you feel good about yourself, can you open up to your partner about these things. And it's also really important for us to understand why our partners sometimes have different sexual interests than we do and how to navigate and communicate about discrepant desires that might emerge. But this all speaks to why it's so necessary to have sound, broadly accessible research to show what's statistically common when it comes to sex.

BEST. SEX. EVER.

What Are the Most Common Kinks in the United States?

Alas, there isn't a lot of research that looks at how *often* folks engage in kinks, but there is a bunch of research that looks at how often folks *fantasize* about certain kinks. For his book, *Tell Me What You Want: The Science of Sexual Desire and How It Can Help You Improve Your Sex Life*, Lehmiller spent two years surveying more than 4,000 Americans from all 50 states about their sexual fantasies. He found that most people had fantasized about at least one kink before.

Below, you'll find a few of the most common kinks folks have fantasized about.

1. BDSM

Bondage and discipline, dominance and submission, sadism, and masochism is the most fantasized-about kink. Lehmiller found that 93 percent of men and 96 percent of women had fantasized about some aspect of BDSM before. BDSM reflects a broad spectrum of behaviors, from mild to wild, and most people fall at the milder end, with fantasies about taking on dominant or submissive roles, like tying up a partner or being tied up and engaging in light sadomasochism (think spanking and biting).

2. Bodily Fluids

Many people reported fantasies in which specific bodily fluids played a big role. Unsurprisingly, male and female ejaculate (i.e., cum and squirt) were the most common. However, other bodily fluids appeared too.

- *45 percent of men and 35 percent of women had fantasies involving spit.*
- *31 percent of men and 14 percent of women had fantasies involving breast milk.*
- *32 percent of men and 15 percent of women had fantasies involving urine.*
- *6 percent of men and 2 percent of women had fantasies involving feces.*

3. Voyeurism

Sixty percent of the participants reported having fantasized about watching someone else undress or have sex. Voyeurism is appealing because we are very visual creatures—it's sort of like watching real-life porn. However, voyeurism fantasies often involve sneaking around too, so part of the appeal might be the thrill of doing something you're not supposed to.

4. Exhibitionism

A lot of people fantasize about putting on a show. Specifically, 42 percent of participants reported having a fantasy about publicly exposing themselves or having sex in front of an audience.

5. Gender Play

A lot of cisgender people use their fantasies as a way of exploring their gender role or expression. Lehmiller found that about 1 in 4 cisgender people had fantasized about cross-dressing, while about 1 in 3 had fantasized about trading bodies with someone of another sex.

These fantasies are sometimes about a desire to break free of traditional gender roles or to explore the self; however, there was also a lot of overlap with BDSM. Several men reported what's commonly referred to as "forced feminization" fantasies, in which a partner "forces" them to dress in traditionally feminine clothing.

6. Cuckolding

Fantasies about watching your partner have sex with someone else are very common, with 58 percent of men and 33 percent of women having fantasized about this before. For some, cuckolding is about self-enhancement—knowing that other people find their partner to be hot actually boosts their self-esteem. For others, it's about wanting to see their partner sexually satisfied—they take pleasure in their partner's pleasure. And for others, there's a BDSM element; often the watcher takes on a submissive role, getting humiliated in the process.

Pro Tip: ➡ Have a Safe Word

You should always have a safe word. Period. You can't predict what you're going to feel during sex, especially when trying something new. Not to mention that there are severe physical dangers when engaging in some kinks, such as impact play (e.g., spanking, flogging, whipping), shibari (Japanese rope bondage), and breath play (i.e., choking). So you need a word that lets your partner know everything needs to stop. A common form of safe word is to say "yellow" when you're getting close to reaching your limit and "red" when it's a hard stop and all sexual activity needs to cease immediately.

KINKS AND FETISHES

How Do I Talk to My Partner About My Kinks or Fetishes?

Whenever you're sharing any fringe sexual desire it's normal to have a fear of rejection. *What if they think I'm a pervert or psychologically damaged?* The truth is, if they think those things, then they're not right for you. You want to be with someone who doesn't shame you for your kinks. That doesn't mean they have to share the same desires; they simply need to accept yours. But how do you even begin to talk to your partner about your kinks? Let's break it down.

Have a conversation outside the bedroom.
When it comes to discussing anything sexual with your partner, it's best to do so when you're clothed—not in the heat of the moment. We have a lot of emotions and thoughts running through our heads when we're about to have sex that can cause us to say (or respond with) inappropriate things. So bring it up the next time you two are casually hanging, like watching Netflix together.

Use a source of media as an introduction to the conversation.
It's always a safe bet to bring up an article, book, or video as a talking point. You can say, "I just read this interesting article about kinks and want to get your thoughts!"

"Start low and go slow."
In other words, start on the more vanilla end of the spectrum when initially revealing your kinks. "When it comes to engaging in sexual self-disclosure, it works the best when it's a gradual process," Lehmiller says. "It gives

you time for trust and intimacy to build, which is necessary when sharing something that a lot of people might not be familiar with."

Ask them about their kinks too.

This should be a conversation, not a monologue. Odds are, they have specific kinks and fantasies they haven't shared with you. Who knows? You two may actually have compatible kinks. So after sharing a milder kink of yours, ask your partner, "What are some things you're into?"

Don't wait too long to share your kinks.

"I've heard of a lot of people who have hidden their kinks from their spouses for decades, and then when it's finally discovered later on, it becomes this major source of conflict—one person feels like they were lied to or deceived," Lehmiller says. "Not to mention that the kinky person was hiding an element of their sexuality for a big chunk of their life, which is a shame." So perhaps wait a couple of months, as opposed to years, to confide in your partner that you'd like to try something on the kinkier end of the spectrum.

Say What Now?

What's a *Switch*?

In the bedroom, some people find they're exclusively dominant or submissive. A *switch* is someone who enjoys being both dominant and submissive. So in one instance, a switch can be the dominant "daddy" or "master." They're the one doing the spanking and choking and tying up their partner. But with another partner, a switch can enjoy being the "baby" or "slave," where they're the one listening to the commands—licking the boot, both literally and metaphorically.

KINKS AND FETISHES

How Do I Bring Kink Into the Boudoir?

It doesn't matter what you're doing—if you do it the same way every time, you're going to get bored. This is true even of sex! That's where kink comes in handy. Kink can help reinvigorate your sex life and get you as excited about the prospect of having sex as when you were a teenager. This is particularly helpful if you're in a monogamous relationship and you've been sleeping with the same person for years on end. So don't think of kink as being "intimidating" or "too intense"—think of it as a tool for reconnecting with your partner sexually (which will likely positively impact *other* aspects of your relationship).

Below are a few ways to incorporate kink in the bedroom, just in case you want to dabble in stepping outside the vanilla box.

Get verbal.

Sex should be loud. You should grunt, moan, and say "fuck yes" at the top of your lungs. It's a time to let go and experience pleasure. But in addition to making noise, you can explore getting verbal with your partner by calling each other names like *daddy/baby* or *sir/madam* (see page 33 for more ideas). You can also explore more derogatory words, like *bitch*, *slut*, *cum dump*, and so on. Of course, talk to your partner first to see which words they want to be called before telling them they're "daddy's good little whore." You'll notice that saying these words or just moaning louder (which is such a small, simple thing you can do) can really enhance your pleasure.

Try out role play.

Here's the thing about role play: You have to give it 100 percent. If you half-ass it, it's not going to work, but if you're able to fully suspend belief, it can pay off big-time. Many popular roles (boss/secretary, teacher/student, stripper/customer) incorporate elements of power and control, where one person is at the mercy of their partner. Exploring these elements can elevate your sex life and naturally create a BDSM dynamic where you get to dominate or be submissive. (Who knows? You and your partner may learn that you *love* this dynamic in the bedroom!)

But it doesn't have to be that serious. Role play can be light and playful, say, if one of you is dressing up as a fox (with ears and a butt plug with a furry tail) and the other is a foxhunter.

Tie each other up.

You can easily tie one another up using things around the house, like ties, silk scarves, and a pair of stockings, or you can purchase a pair of handcuffs, restraints, or bondage rope online. There is a sense of being erotically overwhelmed that comes along with being restrained, and many women [and men] find quite passionate," says Carol Queen, Ph.D., staff sexologist at Good Vibrations, a woman-owned-and-operated sex toy empire. You can tie your partner's hands over their head or tie them to the bed frame. You want to tie them tight enough so that they can't get out but also loose enough not to cause a loss of circulation. You should always have a pair of safety shears handy in case you need to cut your partner out ASAP.

Explore impact play.

Getting spanked, either by a hand, flog, whip, or paddle, sends shock waves throughout your entire body. You feel alert. Your heart starts racing. You wonder when the next jolt of pain is going to come. In short, it makes you feel *alive*.

If you're new to impact play, make sure to start soft and slowly progress to harder (as you check in with your partner). Strike the fleshy parts where there are no vital organs underneath, like the butt, thighs, and back (avoiding the spine). Don't hit on the front side of someone's torso, where the liver, kidneys, heart, lungs, and all those *very* vital organs are.

Deny orgasms.

Right as your partner is getting close to climaxing, pull back and don't let them cum. This will drive them absolutely wild. Then when you finally do let them orgasm, their orgasm will be far stronger than if they came the first time around. Not only does orgasm denial prolong your sexual session, but there's also a playful brattiness that comes with it. ("Uh-uh! You don't get to cum yet!")

BEST. SEX. EVER.

YES/NO/MAYBE?

If the prospect of asking someone to try out a new kink makes your chest tight and palms clammy, we've got your back. Here's what you're going to do: Sit down with your partner and show them this page in the book. (Howdy, partner!) For each kinky item on the list below, you can each say yes, no, or maybe to indicate how open you are to trying it. If either or both of you say no to something, move right along! If you both say maybe—or one person says maybe and one says yes—you can talk about and research it more. And if you both say yes? Well, I think we all know what you're doing tonight.

Y	N	M		Y	N	M	
☐	☐	☐	Age play[1]	☐	☐	☐	Foot fetishism
☐	☐	☐	Anal fisting	☐	☐	☐	Gagging
☐	☐	☐	Animal play[2]	☐	☐	☐	Group sex
☐	☐	☐	Blindfolds	☐	☐	☐	Hair pulling
☐	☐	☐	Biting	☐	☐	☐	Humiliation
☐	☐	☐	Bodily fluids[3]	☐	☐	☐	Leather
☐	☐	☐	Bondage[4]	☐	☐	☐	Masochism[5]
☐	☐	☐	Breath play	☐	☐	☐	Nipple play
☐	☐	☐	Costumes	☐	☐	☐	Nylons
☐	☐	☐	Chastity belts and cages	☐	☐	☐	Orgasm control[6]
☐	☐	☐	Cock and ball torture	☐	☐	☐	Pet play[7]
☐	☐	☐	Cock worship	☐	☐	☐	Role play of any other kind
☐	☐	☐	Cuckolding	☐	☐	☐	Sadism[8]
☐	☐	☐	Dirty talk	☐	☐	☐	Scratching
☐	☐	☐	Domination and submission	☐	☐	☐	Spanking[9]
☐	☐	☐	Electrostimulation	☐	☐	☐	Sploshing[10]
☐	☐	☐	Enemas	☐	☐	☐	Vaginal fisting
☐	☐	☐	Exhibitionism	☐	☐	☐	Voyeurism
☐	☐	☐	Food and sex	☐	☐	☐	Wax play

1. role-playing different ages than you actually are
2. role-playing an animal
3. such as semen, squirt, spit, and pee
4. handcuffs, ropes, restraints, etc.
5. deriving pleasure from experiencing pain
6. a dominant partner dictating when and/or how the submissive partner is allowed to climax
7. role-playing a pet and owner
8. deriving pleasure from inflicting pain
9. or other forms of impact play, such as flogging or whipping
10. putting "wet and messy" substances—think cake or whipped cream—on your body

KINKS AND FETISHES

We Want to Have a Threesome? Now What?

Threesomes are fucking hot. There's something undeniably arousing about feeling overwhelmingly desired by your partner *and* another person, not to mention that there are certain sexual positions you can pull off with a third.

"However, while having a threesome is one of the most common sexual fantasies there is, it's also the fantasy that is least likely to turn out well when people actually do it," Lehmiller warns.

"It's because we don't have scripts for how to navigate multipartner sex," he explains. "So people walk into the situation not knowing who was supposed to do what and when. This uncertainty element is a huge stumbling block for a lot of people."

This means you can't embark on a threesome willy-nilly. You need to plan it out, because nothing should be a surprise in this experience. There shouldn't be any point where you're thinking, *Whoa…I didn't think we'd be doing this*. To avoid any confusion (and subsequent hurt feelings), you need to communicate with your partner before embarking on this fabulous sexual adventure.

(Oh, and if your relationship isn't on solid ground—say you've been arguing a lot, a partner recently cheated, or you two have clear jealousy issues—then don't have a threesome! That will only make matters worse. It's like when a couple has a baby because they think it'll somehow save their marriage…not a good idea!)

How to Prepare

Talk to your partner about what you want to do.
Do you want to fuck this other person together? Do you just want to kiss? Only watch? Get tied up? Let your partner know how your ideal threesome would pan out and vice versa.

Discuss rules and boundaries.
Do you plan to wear condoms when you have sex? (You should!) Do you only want to do oral? Are they allowed to sleep over after?

Own your "no."
Don't feel guilty or immature for not wanting to engage in a sexual activity. If your partner wants to do something and you're not comfortable with it, make that clear. Don't just go along with it. That's a recipe for disaster.

Discuss with the third.
After you and your partner have decided what you do and don't want to do, talk to the third person about it. Otherwise, how the hell would they know? Also, there's no harm in saying, "This is the first time we've had a threesome, so we're a little nervous." I'd be willing to bet they're a little nervous too. Or if they're a threesome pro, they'll say, "Great! I'm excited to show you the ropes!"

Have a safe word.
You may think you're okay with watching your partner get plowed by another person, but the moment their legs are up in the air, you come to realize: *NOPE, I HATE THIS*. That is totally fine, "but given that you can't predict how you'll respond when having a threesome, it's necessary to have a safe word," Lehmiller says. If you do use the safe word, you can say, "I'm just not into this as much as I thought I was going to be, so we're going to have to call it."

KINKS AND FETISHES

What to Do During

Make sure the threesome doesn't turn into a twosome.
When you're in a threesome, it can be easy to become focused on the third person since you've never had sex with them before and you've already boned your partner a ton. Plus, the third may be more into one person than the other. Even if that's the case, you want to do your best to make sure no one feels excluded. "That doesn't mean that everybody has to be providing equal attention to everyone the entire time," Lehmiller says. That's really impossible. Nevertheless, don't ignore the third; find a balance!

Don't feel pressured to be in every moment.
In a similar vein, if the other two people are involved, don't insert yourself (no pun intended). Let them have their tender moment. Enjoy watching for a little bit before you go back to kissing, touching, and fucking them.

What to Do After

Check in and see how everyone's feeling.
When the third person leaves, you can debrief with your partner to see what they liked and disliked— that way, if you two decide to have another threesome, it'll be even better.

THE BEST ___ EVER

The Best Threesome/Group Sex I've Ever Had

"[It was during] a sex-positive group trip where we rented a villa on the beach for a week. When the sun went down, we would congregate in the living room with blankets and pillows, creating a giant bed on the floor, and play together. Girls' beach-tangled hair blending together as they kissed. Couples with skin golden from the sun undulating as others watched. Mouths, legs, hands, and sex toys everywhere late into the night." —**Natalie, 37**

"My friend and I surprised a female friend of ours with an MMF [bisexual male-male-female threesome] for her birthday. It was early June in an old Victorian hotel in Telluride, Colorado. We covered the bed in lilac blooms and made a night of it." —**Tom, 50**

"An all-guy orgy with four other guys and myself in college. It was completely animalistic with five horny guys all going at it for hours." —**Nate, 43**

"I hooked up with a M-F couple in my 20s. He was bi, and she was cool with that and enjoyed inviting other guys to play. It was wild! Everyone had every hole filled at one point or another. We were in their shared uni accommodation, so trying to be vaguely discreet about it all, but I don't think we succeeded, especially not the second time round...." —**Dave, 37**

"Anytime a couple has asked me to be their third. Being the object of desire for a couple gives me an ego boner." —**Gregg, 30**

KINKS AND FETISHES

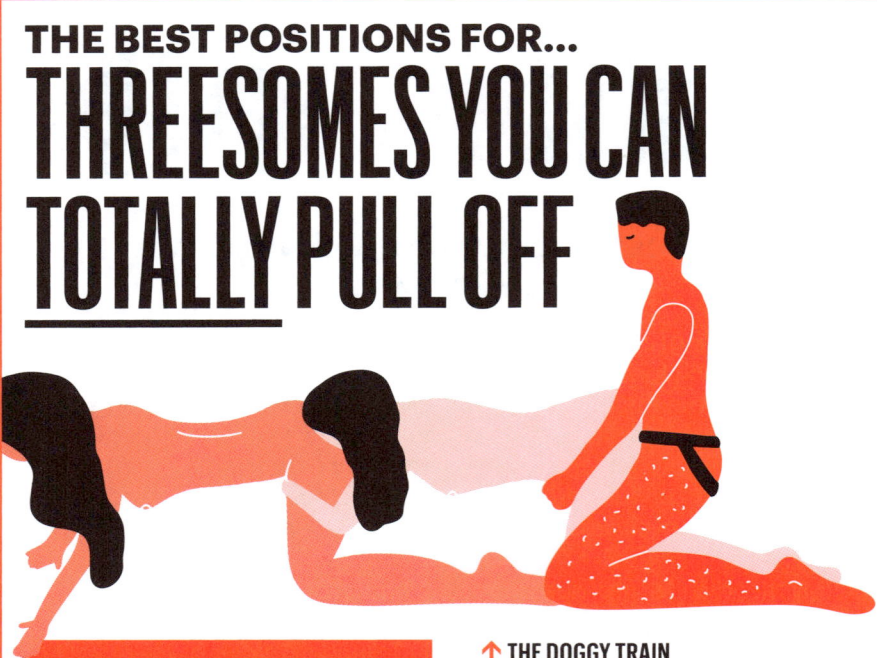

THE BEST POSITIONS FOR...
THREESOMES YOU CAN TOTALLY PULL OFF

To help illustrate these positions, the instructions are given with "you" as a penetrator—but remember, these positions are versatile!

↑ THE DOGGY TRAIN

You're the "caboose" of this train, penetrating your partner in doggy style. The middle partner is then either digitally penetrating or eating out the head of the train, who's also on their knees, bent forward in a classic doggy-style position.

DOUBLE COWGIRL →

While one partner straddles your waist in a traditional cowgirl position, the other straddles your face, allowing you to go down on them. The person sitting on your face can straddle you either way, but it's typically better if they straddle you while facing the other person, so they, too, can kiss and touch one another.

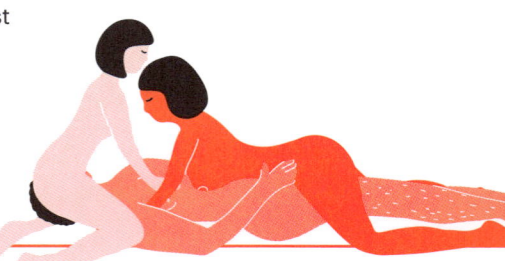

BEST. SEX. EVER.

↓ DOUBLE ORAL

Your two partners are on their knees in front of you, both blowing you at the same time. It's best if one blower focuses on your testicles while the other focuses on your penis. Depending on if you're into it, one partner could actually be on their knees rimming you from behind while the other person goes down on you from the front.

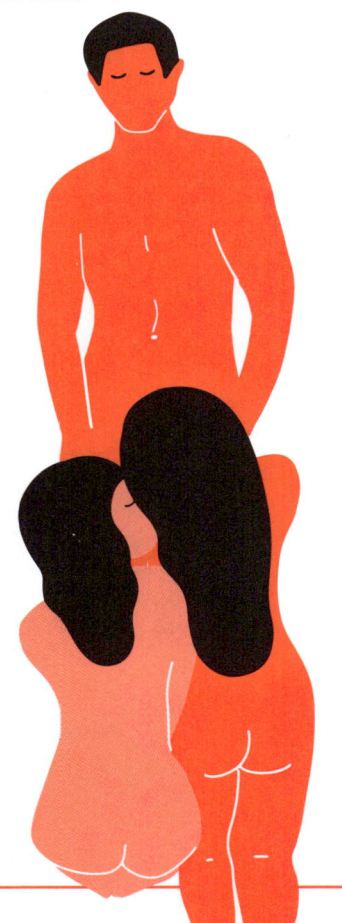

69 TRAIN ↓

Everyone is lying on their sides in a circular position eating out/blowing one another. (FYI, this position can be tough to pull off when people are of drastically different heights.)

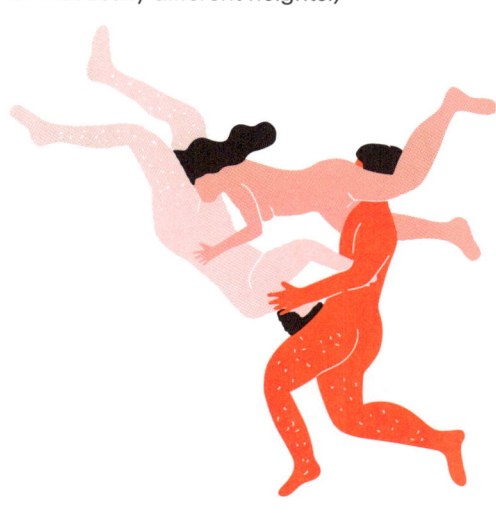

↓ THE DOGGY DELUXE

You're having sex with the first partner in doggy style. The third partner is lying on their back, positioned to allow the middle person to go down on them.

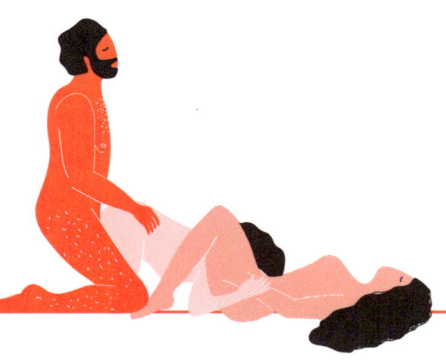

KINKS AND FETISHES

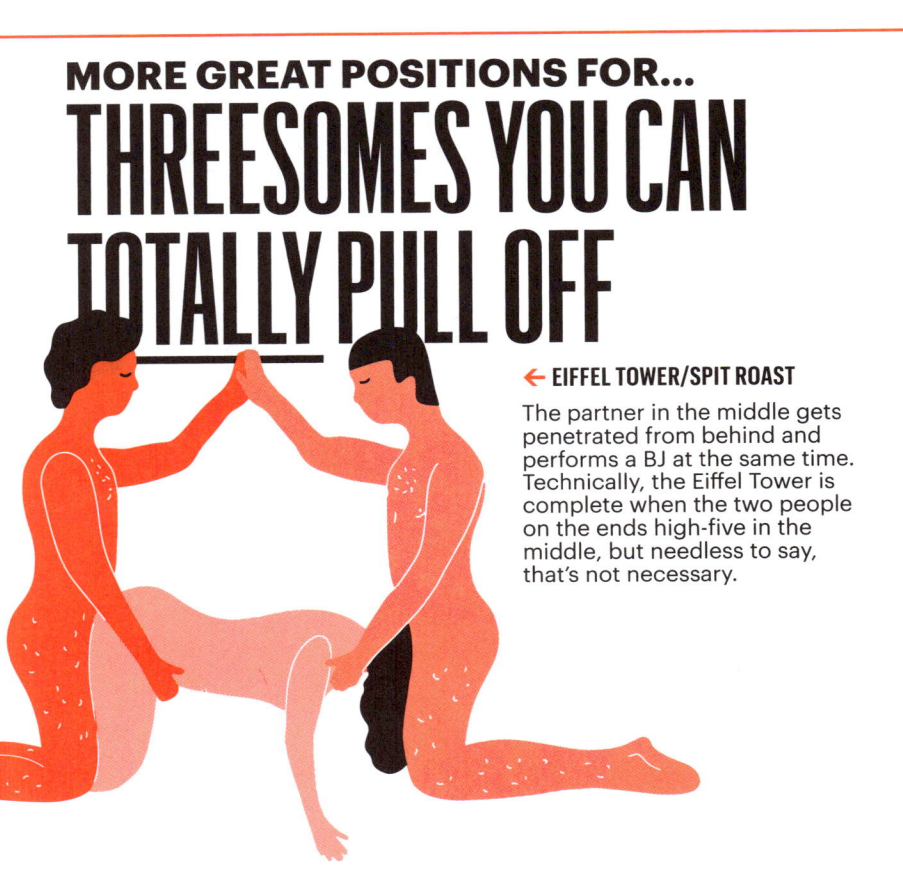

MORE GREAT POSITIONS FOR...
THREESOMES YOU CAN TOTALLY PULL OFF

← EIFFEL TOWER/SPIT ROAST

The partner in the middle gets penetrated from behind and performs a BJ at the same time. Technically, the Eiffel Tower is complete when the two people on the ends high-five in the middle, but needless to say, that's not necessary.

CLASSIC DP (DOUBLE PENETRATION) →

One person lies on their back underneath the vulva-owning partner. The other partner penetrates them from behind. There are variations of DP. You can do one penis in the vagina and one in the anus, two in the vagina, or two in the anus.

BEST. SEX. EVER.

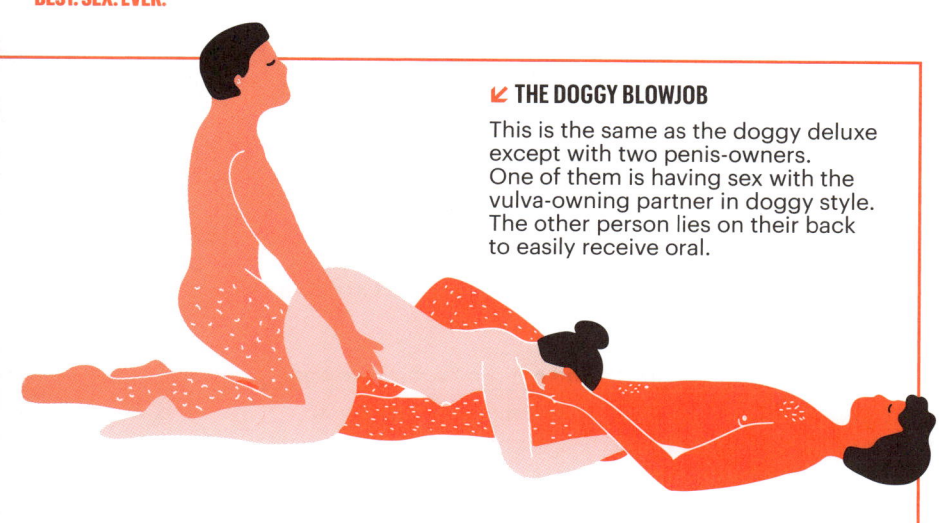

↙ THE DOGGY BLOWJOB

This is the same as the doggy deluxe except with two penis-owners. One of them is having sex with the vulva-owning partner in doggy style. The other person lies on their back to easily receive oral.

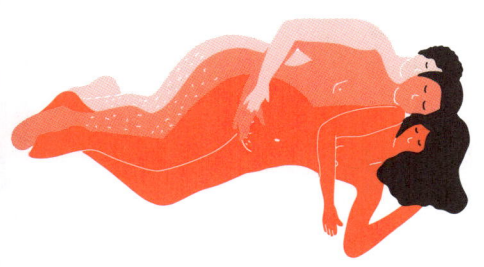

← THE TRAIN (AKA DAISY CHAIN)

Everyone lies on their sides and penetrates the person in front of them either anally or vaginally. Really squish yourselves together for this position. If you have too much space between you, someone is going to slip out.

Say What Now?

What's a *Unicorn*?

A unicorn is a bisexual woman who's down to have a threesome with a male-female couple. Bi women are *constantly* solicited for threesomes on dating apps, and it can be frustrating if they're looking to find a serious partner, or if a straight-identifying couple tries to use them as an "experiment." On the other hand, unicorns, while rare, are totally down to have casual threesomes with couples. (FYI, a male unicorn is called a dragon!)

KINKS AND FETISHES

Sex Party Tips for Newbies

While no two sex parties are the same, we've amassed some universal best practices from personal experience that'll help you succeed in any sex club.

Your first time around, attend a more "social" sex party.

If it's your first time ever attending a sex party, you probably don't want to go to a party where everyone starts fucking the moment they step through the doors. It might help you ease into things by attending a more social party, so you can talk to folks and get to know them before undressing. Many sex clubs have erotic performances or sexy games before the actual sex commences.

Bring a partner in crime.

A number of mixed-gender play parties won't let single men attend by themselves. You need to have a partner with you. Even if they don't mandate having someone, we highly recommend you attend with a partner. That person can be someone you're sleeping with or simply a friend. It can feel a bit awkward walking around by yourself at these parties, and some folks may unwittingly judge you—assuming you're a creep—if you're out on the prowl by yourself.

Also, sex is not guaranteed at these parties. By going with someone you're sexual with, there's a better chance you'll get laid, both by your partner and by others.

Set personal boundaries before attending.

Think about what you want to do before you go to the sex party. It's easy to get "swept up" in the moment and do something that you later regret. Don't feel pressured to do it all your first night. There will *always* be more sex parties.

Set boundaries with your partner before attending.

If you're hitting up a party with an existing sexual partner, then you need to have a conversation about what you're allowed to do sexually. Are you two allowed to have sex with other people independently or only as a unit? Or would you rather not have sex at all and just take in the scene? There are no wrong answers—it's simply whatever agreement you and your partner make.

Wear something that makes you feel sexy.

Do you know who's no fun? The guy who goes to a sex party in a frumpy T-shirt and jeans. Whether it's a harness, collar, or goddamn jockstrap, wear something that makes you feel empowered and sexy. Additionally, most sex parties have a dress code. If they do, follow it.

Be friendly and direct.

There's no need for corny pickup lines at sex parties. You can go up to someone you're attracted to, introduce yourself with a smile, and ask how their night is going. It will become very clear if they're interested in talking to you or not. If they reply, "My night's going better now," or "I was bored until you came along," it's a good sign they want to bang. If they respond, "It's going fine," and are looking around the room for someone else, then simply reply, "Same here. Great to meet you," and walk the hell away.

Get enthusiastic consent for all sexual behaviors.

Consent is required for all sexual activity—and yes, that includes at a party where the express purpose is having sex. When you go to a sex party, you need to get a verbal yes before engaging in any sexual behavior. Remember, you can ask for consent in sexy ways: "God, I really want to kiss you right now. Can I?"

KINKS AND FETISHES

Don't be afraid to say, "Not interested."
There may be folks who want to have sex with you, and you might not be interested. Totally fine! There's no easier place to reject someone than at a sex party. You can always say, "I'm not looking to play right now," or "I just want to have sex with my partner tonight." After rejecting them, just walk away. You can say, "I'm going to find my friend." If a person begins to harass or follow you, speak to someone working the event. They will help you.

CONFESSIONS

"My Most Awkward Group Sex Experience Was…"

"An ex-girlfriend walked in on me and a buddy having sex. I had told her I was bi, but she didn't believe me. After watching dumbstruck for a minute or so, she made her presence known by stripping down and trying to join us. My buddy and I were caught off guard at first, but it turned into a fun night." **—Nate, 43**

"I unicorned for a couple that spent the whole time looking deeply into each other's eyes—ignoring me—saying, 'You know I love you more than anything, right, babe?'" **—Natalie, 37**

"The couple got into a physical altercation while I got dressed, so I had to run out of their house!" **—Gregg, 30**

BEST. SEX. EVER.

SEXPLAIN IT

Dear Sexplain It,

I'm worried I'm too kinky and I'm never going to find someone. I've tried to share some of my kinks with my partners before, but they always get weirded out and we end up breaking up. I have some pretty typical kinks (BDSM, spanking, etc.) but then I also have kinks that fall into the raunchy and even taboo category. I can sometimes find someone I like who is interested in the same kink but only for a casual hookup. Never to date. I'm worried this means I'm going to be single forever. How can I find someone who is into the same stuff I am and wants a long-term thing?

—*Kinky in Florida*

Dear Kinky in Florida,

I can say with certainty there are plenty of people out there who have your kinks, no matter how "out there" they may be. But I get why you're having a hard time. Achieving a fulfilling long-term relationship isn't just a matter of finding someone with compatible kinks. You also want someone smart, caring, attractive, and all that other shit.

I have a question for you: Are you active in your local kink scene? "Many cities have sex and BDSM clubs and dungeons where like-minded people gather to play," says sex and relationship expert Shamyra Howard, L.C.S.W.

KINKS AND FETISHES

And if you haven't already, I'd search for a partner on FetLife or Recon. These are social networks for kinky people looking to connect meaningfully—not just hook up.

With these apps, you won't struggle with "Am I too kinky for them?" or "How do I let them know I like to be [insert your kink] without freaking them out?" You say what you're into and you search for other folks who are into the same things. Bada bing, bada boom. No shame. No judgment.

If you've already been trying and failing to connect with other people in the kink community, then maybe you need to adjust what you're looking for.

Your question is no longer "Where can I find an ideal mate who shares every single one of my particular kinks?" It's "Where can I find an ideal mate who empowers me to indulge in my specific kinks in a way that suits us both?" Enter the open relationship.

"If you connect with someone who is not interested in participating in the same kinks as you, simply find out if it's mutually acceptable for you to have a kink partner," Howard says. With a kink partner, you'll be able to get your sexual needs met. So, I would write that you're seeking an open relationship in your dating profile, if you use dating apps.

Here's your to-do list: Get on the kinky social networking sites, add that you're looking for an open relationship on your dating app bios, and widen your search for partners so that you're looking for a romantic partner *and* a kink partner. This way, you can have your cake and eat it too.

BEST. SEX. EVER.

CHAPTER 7

SELF-LOVE

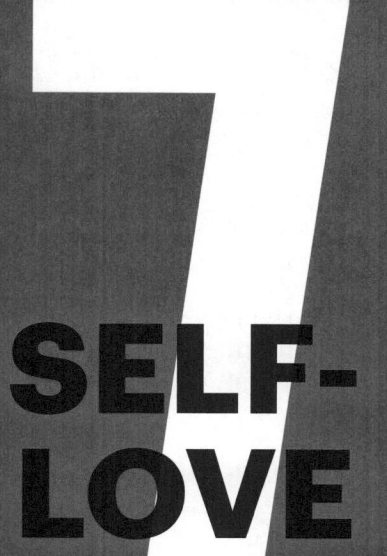

YOUR SEXPERT

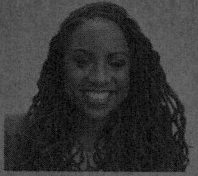

Sexologist and *Men's Health* advisory panel member **Shamyra Howard, L.C.S.W.**, is the author of the book *Use Your Mouth*.

There's a good chance you're still jerking off the same way you did when you were 13 years old: with just your hand and as quickly as possible. *Boring!* Here's how to forever change your solo *and* partnered sex life.

SELF-LOVE

How Do I Step Up My Masturbation Game?

Why should anyone even care about masturbation?
HOWARD: Masturbation is essential. First off, it's one of the first ways we learn about our bodies and pleasure. But even as we age, it's important because it helps us learn our likes and dislikes by connecting us more to our bodies. Besides, pleasure is our birthright. We all deserve it. So why not?

Can solo masturbation potentially harm your sex life with a partner?
Well, it can be either a detriment or a benefit. It becomes a detriment when it impedes your sexual activity or ability to have sexual intimacy. And that happens because we don't masturbate the way we have sex. So if you're gripping too hard when you masturbate (which is common among many [cis] men), you may not be able to orgasm when with a partner because you've sensitized your body to need an amount of pressure that no vagina or anus can give.

So how can masturbating be a positive influence in your sex life?
As long as you're switching things up when you masturbate, you get an opportunity to explore and try different things with your body and to learn what you like. You can learn how you like your penis touched, which things turn you on, and which angles lead to more pleasure. All that stuff.

Is there something specific you should focus on while masturbating?

Everybody likes something different, but three main things guys can focus on are texture, temperature, and pressure. Focusing on these sensations during sex, instead of focusing on all your worries (or about whether you'll orgasm), is called "sensate focus." By focusing on our bodily senses, we can get out of our heads and enjoy the masturbatory experience more. And if we have this sensate focus during sex with a partner, we can enhance our sexual experience with that partner too.

What do most cis guys get wrong when masturbating?

Well, that's the thing. Many guys are masturbating the same way they did when they were teens—all rushed. You need to change things up. If you're right-handed, use your left hand; involve sex toys; or try masturbating on your stomach. Also, don't focus only on your genitals. You have a whole body. Get your nipples, perineum, and anus involved. And don't focus solely on the orgasm! Most people masturbate because they want that release, but allow yourself to focus on the moment of intimacy between you and yourself.

SELF-LOVE

What Are New Ways to Masturbate?

Most people with a penis learn to masturbate as quickly and quietly as possible. After all, when you're a testosterone-loaded adolescent, you have to contend with the very real risk of your parents or siblings walking in and disturbing your, *uh*, personal time.

But if you've been jerking off the same way since you were a teenager, it's high time to switch it up. It won't just make your masturbatory experience more pleasurable—you may also learn a thing or two that can translate to when you're having sex with a partner. (Uchenna "UC" Ossai, Pelvic PT certified sexuality counselor, sex expert Emily Morse, and NYU professor of Human Sexuality Zhana Vrangalova, Ph.D. contributed these fun tips to *Men's Health*.)

Change the position you masturbate in.

You've likely masturbated in the same position for years now, so try switching it up. If you are a stander, try lying on your back. Maybe put your feet against the wall or up behind you. If you do it at your desk, do it on your bed. Do it facedown and rub your dick against your sheets. Plus, changing positioning can improve your pelvic-floor muscle resting tone, which can help improve the blood flow to your penis. So changing up your masturbation positions not only feels pleasurable for the novelty but may also increase the strength of your erections. Win-win, baby!

Don't ignore the taint (perineum).

The perineum is the strip of skin between your testicles and anus. It's filled with very sensitive nerve endings, so it feels pleasurable when touched.

Next time you masturbate, try pressing a vibrator—any vibrator that is easy to grip and gives strong vibrations—to your perineum while stroking your penis with your other hand. There are also prostate massagers that stimulate the perineum too, if you want to get your anus involved.

Switch up your grip and speed of stroking.

Have you ever heard of the "death grip"? If you find yourself having a hard time reaching orgasm during sex with a partner, it might be because you're squeezing your penis too hard and stroking too fast while masturbating. To prevent this, make sure you switch up the grip and stroking speed (i.e., use less pressure and stroke slower) so you're used to having an orgasm in different ways.

Switch hands.

You've probably tried incorporating your nondominant hand into your solo act. You may have even attempted the mythical "stranger"—sitting on your hand until it falls asleep and then using it to simulate the sensation of someone else doing the dirty work. But you can also use your opposite hand in more creative ways.

Turn your hand so it slides down your penis forefinger-first, and twist it as you stroke. You could also try holding your penis against your stomach with one hand while rapidly sliding a few fingers up and down the underside of your shaft.

Try edging.

The three-minute speed jerk is fine most days. But if you have a little extra time, edging—also called the stop-and-start method—can help you achieve more intense orgasms. (See page 82 for more on edging.)

Work yourself right up to the edge of ejaculation, then take a short break—just enough time for your erection to soften a bit. Then start the process over again. Do

SELF-LOVE

this three or four times before you ejaculate and you'll experience stronger orgasms.

Use a masturbation sleeve.

Sex toys aren't just for people with a vulva. For penis-owners, you can use a masturbation sleeve, like a Fleshlight, the popular handheld column that you slip over your junk to simulate the feel of real vaginal or anal sex. The inside materials of the column vary from brand to brand, but they're usually made from some form of soft silicone or adjacent material.

Use a vibrator for your penis.

Vibrators have traditionally been marketed to people with a vulva, which makes sense, given that most vulva-owners need some form of external clitoral stimulation to climax during penetrative sex. But in recent years, there's been an increase in vibrating sex toys designed for dicks because those vibrations can feel fantastic on penises too! One 2012 study found that 44 percent of heterosexual cis men had enjoyed the experience of using a vibrator at some point in their life. Our advice: Don't be shy about trying some of these toys.

Bring your balls into the mix.

There are almost as many sex-specific nerve endings in your testicles as there are in your penis. Don't neglect them! While individual preferences and sensitivities play a big role in what you'll enjoy, a lot of men discover an untapped source of stimulation—and more intense orgasms—by pulling down on their testicles rhythmically before ejaculation. (Another good use of your less dominant hand!)

BEST. SEX. EVER.

HOW DO I KNOW IF I'M <u>ADDICTED TO PORN?</u>

Well, the entire concept of porn addiction is up for debate in the medical community. To be honest, it really seems like a matter of semantics, and frankly, it doesn't matter if it "technically" qualifies as an addiction. Porn is awesome—but you want to make sure it isn't negatively impacting other aspects of your life, Howard says.

Below is a checklist to give you a sense of if you're "addicted" to porn. (This checklist can't diagnose anything, but if you find yourself relating to some of the items on the list, consider talking to a therapist.)

- [ ] **Are you watching porn at work?**
- [ ] **Do you watch porn to distract yourself from how you're feeling?**
- [ ] **Are you unable to orgasm without watching porn?**
- [ ] **Do you get anxious when you're in a situation where you can't watch porn?**
- [ ] **Are you late to set plans because you're watching porn?**
- [ ] **Do you cancel set plans because you're watching porn?**
- [ ] **Are you unable to get erect with a partner?**
- [ ] **Are you unable to orgasm with a partner?**
- [ ] **Do you shut your eyes and imagine you're watching porn when you're with a partner?**
- [ ] **Has your porn consumption put a strain on your relationship with your partner?**
- [ ] **Has anyone in your life ever said you have a problem with your porn consumption?**

SELF-LOVE

What Are the Health Benefits of Masturbating?

If masturbation *just* satisfied our sexual urges, it would be enough. If it *just* helped us embrace our fantasies, it would be enough. If it *just* led to orgasm, it would be enough. But it *also* has health benefits that have nothing to do with arousal and pleasure.

Did you know masturbation can:

Lower your risk of prostate cancer.

A 2004 study found that cis men who ejaculated more than 21 times a month reduced their risk of prostate cancer by roughly 33 percent, compared with guys who did the deed only four to seven times a month. In 2016, researchers followed up with that same group of guys from 2004 and found that those who ejaculated eight to 12 times per month reduced their prostate cancer risk by 10 percent. Masturbation is out here literally saving lives.

Help you de-stress and improve your mood.

Masturbating and ejaculation release a bunch of feel-good neurochemicals like dopamine, serotonin, oxytocin, and endorphins. These chemicals can lift your spirits and activate the reward circuits in your brain. So if you're in a bad mood or you're feeling overwhelmed, give yourself a quick yank to recalibrate.

Aid you in falling asleep.

Before you reach for that melatonin (or get a prescription), try masturbating before you go to bed. Masturbating and ejaculation release prolactin, the "roll over and fall asleep" hormone. It's why you often want to pass out after having sex. No, you don't release as much prolactin masturbating as you do having sex—your brain does know the difference—but you still should release enough to help aid in those nighttime z's.

Keep you nice and hard for years to come.

You know the phrase, "If you don't use it, you lose it?" Well, that goes for you penis too. As you age, you naturally lose muscle tone—yup, even down there.

Masturbation "keeps the angle of your dangle perky," says clinical sexologist Gloria Brame, Ph.D. That's because the smooth muscle of your penis needs to be enriched with oxygen, which is delivered whenever there's a rush of blood to your member (i.e., when you get an erection).

Delay ejaculation when you're with a partner.

If you never masturbated, you would bust so goddamn quickly every time you had sex! Just think of the buildup. But also, you can learn which parts of your penis are sensitive and train your body to last longer with techniques like edging (see page 82).

Pro Tip: ➡ Lubes to Use in a Pinch

When you jack off without any lubrication, you run the risk of chafing your penis, especially if you're circumcised. Not to mention that jacking off with lube just feels better. But sometimes you don't have any lube lying around the house. Lucky for you, there are a bunch of household items you can use as a substitute. Vaseline, olive oil, coconut oil, and aloe vera are all great lube alternatives. They are body-safe and provide maximum lubrication. One note: oils can stain your sheets, so we recommend putting a towel down if you plan to masturbate with them.

SELF-LOVE

Why Do I Need to Try Mutual Masturbation?

Mutual masturbation is underutilized, underappreciated, and underfunded! (Okay, that last part isn't true, but it's a fact that most people don't engage in mutual masturbation with their partners nearly enough!)

There's this idea that mutual masturbation isn't "sex" because there's no penetration, "but sex is so much more than penetration," Howard explains. "Sex is any type of emotional, spiritual, physical, or erotic connection, and that includes mutual masturbation."

So here are a few reasons you *need* to try mutual masturbation ASAP.

You'll learn how your partner touches themselves.

You may notice that your partner lightly touches their clitoris or they go to town on it with a vibrator on full blast. Maybe they touch their clit in circles or they go up and down or they ignore the clit for deep vaginal penetration. Whatever it is that they're doing, learn from it so that the next time you're fingering them, you can copy their movements to give them exactly what they want.

Because you're tired AF but you still want to get off together.

The truth is, sometimes you're not in the mood for penetrative sex. You had a long-ass day and are tired, but you still want to get off. Or in the case of many queer men, you *are* in the mood but you're not clean down there, so no anal for you! That doesn't mean you two can't do something sexual; it just means you can't stick it in his butt. Enter mutual masturbation. It's a way to be sexual with one another and connect without putting in all the work (or douching).

You can watch porn together.

Watching porn with your partner can be a hella erotic experience. You get to embrace elements of your fantasies. You get to see what turns your partner on. And you get some ideas for new things to try out when you two go back to having oral and penetrative sex.

Because sometimes, only *your* hand will do.

We've all been there. You're having sex with someone and it's sublime, but you just can't finish. You have to do it your damn self to get the job done. Well, with mutual masturbation, you two can do just that.

SELF-LOVE

THE BUYER$ GUIDE TO...
<u>PENIS</u> TOYS

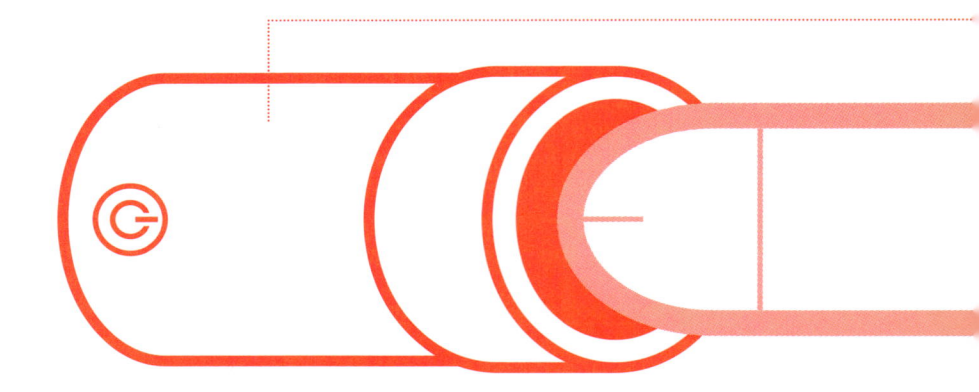

Anal and prostate toys got covered on page 108, so they are not covered here. But PSA: You *absolutely* can use prostate massagers, butt plugs, and anal beads while masturbating. In fact, we recommend you try them out alone before using them with a partner so that you can familiarize yourself with the sensation. Here are some prime penis-centric toys ideal for masturbation.

BEST. SEX. EVER.

MASTURBATION SLEEVES (aka male masturbators) come in many shapes and forms, but they're something you place over your penis to jerk off with. There are sleeves like the Fleshlight that look like a vulva or anus (or are molded from a famous porn star), but then there are sleeves from brands like Tenga that look like modern art sculptures. Some sleeves vibrate, whereas others have a mechanism in the device that simulates being jerked off or given a blowjob.

COCK RINGS may be thought of as a couples toy, but you can absolutely use them during solo sex time. A vibrating cock ring enhances your pleasure, making you more likely to experience a full-body orgasm instead of one localized to your genitals.

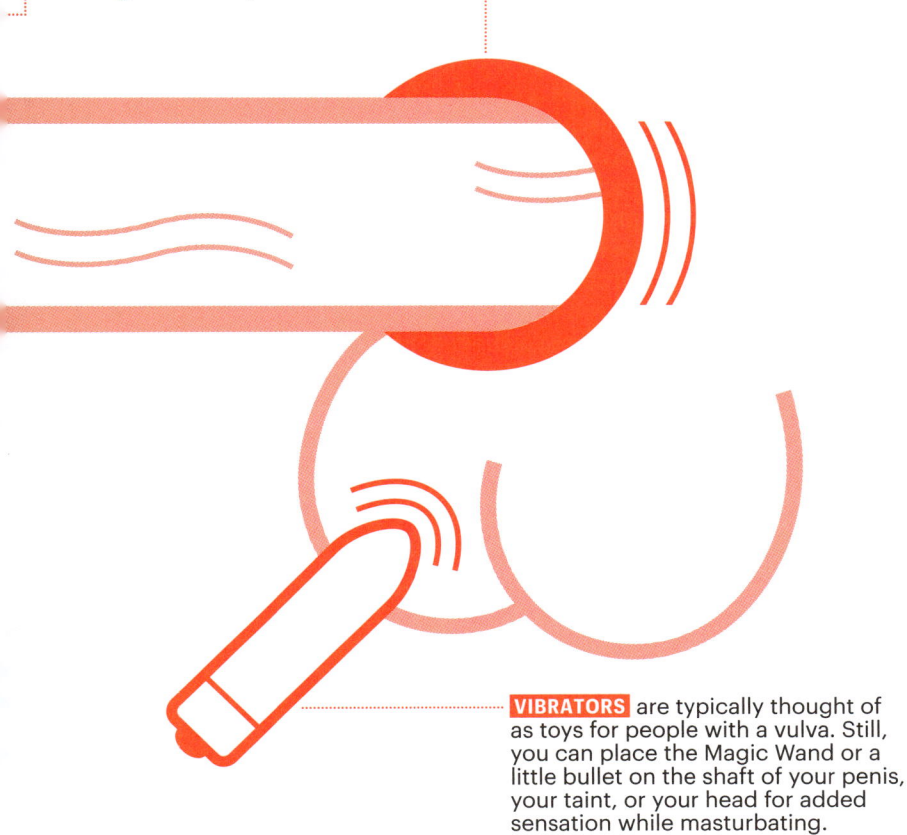

VIBRATORS are typically thought of as toys for people with a vulva. Still, you can place the Magic Wand or a little bullet on the shaft of your penis, your taint, or your head for added sensation while masturbating.

SELF-LOVE

Can I Masturbate Too Much?

Yes, you can—just like you can do *anything* too much. You can work out too much. You can eat too much. You can even *read* too much. But as with anything that becomes "too much," it becomes an issue only when it starts causing issues in other areas of your life.

So if you're masturbating three times a day—once in the morning when you wake up, once when you get home from work, and once before going to bed—that's likely not a problem. Why? Because you're still getting your work done, seeing friends, and living your best life. "Now, if you're late to work because you're masturbating in the morning, that's a problem," Howard says. "If you can't complete a task without masturbating, that's a problem." So too is it a problem if you can't get hard with your partner because you've been jerking off all day. "It comes down to this: Are you having any negative consequences because of your masturbation habits? If so, it's an indicator you might have an issue and want to cut back."

Pro Tip: ➡ Consider Masturbating After a Workout

Do you ever feel *really* horny after working out? Well, there's a reason for that. You release hormones while working out, including adrenaline and dopamine. It's excellent to masturbate after working out because your endorphins are high and blood flow is great. Not to mention that it's a great reward for kicking ass at the gym.

What Are the Biggest Myths Porn Perpetuates?

When asked, "What are some things porn would have you believe about sex that aren't true?" Howard was quick to reply, "All of it."

"Porn is for eroticization, not education," Howard says. It's arousing as all hell to watch. You can pick up a thing or two you may want to try out. But outside of that, you shouldn't think that porn is in any way "real." Here are a few of the ways porn creates unrealistic expectations.

Everyone stays hard the whole time.

Here's what you don't see when watching porn: the Viagra they took beforehand (or the Trimix they injected directly into their dick). And when the guy does get soft because meds aren't working, do you know what they do? They take a break until they can get hard again. Oh, and not to ruin the fantasy even more, but often porn stars look at porn while they're doing the money shot on someone's face. (That's the only way they can get off!)

Penises are always big.

"Porn would have you think that every guy has a huge nine-inch penis, but that's just not true. Not to mention that they film from angles to make someone's penis look even bigger," Howard says.

There aren't condoms.

Where are the condoms? Nowhere to be found (unless you're watching amateur porn). And that's because people don't *like* watching porn with condoms. That's all fine and dandy for the performers who get STI-tested before shooting, but if you want to prevent STI transmission and unwanted pregnancy, then you should definitely roll one on.

No one uses lube.

Lube is a must, *especially* when doing anal. (Refer back to Chapter 5.) Yet in porn, there isn't a bottle of lube to be found. (Of course they use it, but you never see them applying or reapplying!)

The lack of cleaning between anal and vaginal penetration.

A surefire way to give your partner a UTI? Going straight from anal to vaginal sex without washing your dick off first. Bacteria (yes, from poop) get transferred into the vagina, and that can cause a UTI.

All sex is rough sex.

Sex can be intimate, loving, and tender. While this may sound obvious, it doesn't describe the majority of what you'll find on a mainstream tube site like Pornhub. It's a lot of hair pulling, face slapping, throat fucking, and jackhammering. Don't get us wrong, all that hardcore sex can be highly arousing, but not everyone is into it. More importantly, it shouldn't be the gold standard for sex.

Every cis woman squirts.

Modern studies estimate that between 10 and 54 percent of vulva-owners can squirt. (Yes, quite a wide range, but this hasn't been studied in *that* much detail.) And according to a 2013 study of 320 participants, the amount of "squirt" (i.e., ejaculate) released ranges from 0.3 milliliters to more than 150 milliliters. That's anything from a few drops to half a cup. Still, even if a person *does* squirt, they don't necessarily squirt every time and they're (likely) not shooting liquid across the room.

No awkward moments.

"We fall off the bed. We queef. We pass gas. We bleed. We accidentally kick our partner in the face," Howard says. "None of this is depicted in porn." To that end, you don't get to see the laughter and joy in porn. It's all so intense. You can make jokes while boning. After all, sex, first and foremost, should be *fun*!

Say What Now?

What's *Ethical Porn*?

Ethical porn (sometimes called *feminist porn* or *fair trade porn*) is pornography that focuses on the well-being of the performers. Ethical porn makes sure that all performers are getting a fair rate, are treated with respect, and are doing things only within their comfort zone.

Often ethical porn breaks the mold from more mainstream porn by focusing on female pleasure, picturing all body types, and showcasing queer love. That said, ethical porn doesn't have anything to do with the intensity, kinkiness, or roughness of the sexual acts. It can be rough and raunchy as all hell as long as the performers are treated with respect and getting paid fairly for their work!

SELF-LOVE

SEXPLAIN IT

Dear Sexplain It,

I've been with my boyfriend for about two years now, and up until recently, everything has been great. We get along really well and have sex a few times a week. We totally trust each other, except for this one thing that's been bugging me lately.

I found out my boyfriend receives a lot of nudes from guys on Instagram and Snapchat, both unsolicited and solicited. When I caught him in the act, I told him I felt weird about it. He said it was a recent thing he started doing. Sometimes he looks at them when he masturbates, but that's it. He said it's no different from porn, and it's not like he's planning on cheating on me with any of these guys. Obviously, I don't care if he looks at porn—we often watch porn together. But this feels different.

I'm a little suspicious, but I don't know if I'm jealous for no real reason. Am I overreacting, or is our relationship in trouble?

—Trouble in Paradise

Dear Trouble in Paradise,

Overreacting means having an unreasonably over-the-top response to something relatively benign. You are not overreacting. (In fact, I think you're acting pretty chill about this, TBH.)

You've just learned that your partner asks other men to send him nudes and he masturbates to them. You're uncomfortable, and you're concerned about the future of your relationship—and rightfully so! Your partner didn't tell you himself about his new passion for collecting nudes from thirsty gays. Lord knows he easily could have.

Instead, you caught him in the act. His omission of the truth—or lie, depending on your moral compass—proves that he was hiding something. So it makes sense that you still feel uneasy, even after talking to him about it.

I showed your message to psychotherapist Daryl Appleton, L.M.H.C., and she seemed concerned about your boyfriend's dismissive attitude. "The red flag I see has less to do with viewing and getting nudes and more in the potential brush-off you received from your partner," Appleton says. "While it doesn't sound like he is cheating on you, it does sound like he did not validate your feelings around the situation."

And for the record, your boyfriend's claim that receiving nudes is the same as watching porn is total bullshit. When you watch porn, you're not engaging with the performers on the screen. When you're soliciting nudes, you're actually messaging back and forth with someone— not to mention that the guy sending nudes is likely asking for your boyfriend to reciprocate with nudes of his own. That's the etiquette.

And even if your boyfriend says he doesn't plan on cheating on you with these people, the possibility is still there. These guys could send your boyfriend their addresses. That shit doesn't happen with porn, and I bet that's why he likes getting nudes: because it is so clearly different from watching porn.

SELF-LOVE

So is your relationship in trouble? Yes, but you can fix it—as long as your partner is down to put the work in too. First things first, address that he dismissed you. I'd also see if your boyfriend is unknowingly dealing with a bigger issue—in other words, maybe he's not aware that getting nudes is fulfilling some deeper need. Perhaps he isn't satisfied sexually? He hasn't felt connected to you lately? Something else?

To get to the bottom of *all* this, try saying: "I know we previously spoke about this, but I still feel really uncomfortable knowing that you're receiving nudes. I know you said it's just like porn, but to me, it's not, since you're actually talking and engaging with these men. It makes me worried that you're not satisfied with our relationship and you're looking for other men to be with. I'm having a hard time trusting you and believing that everything is fine between us. And I would like us to get back on the same page. Can we talk about it?"

The best-case scenario is that he stops with the nudes because they make you uncomfortable and he opens up about how he's been feeling lately. The worst-case scenario is that he doubles down, saying everything is fine and that receiving nudes is no indication of any larger problem in your relationship. In which case...fuck this dude. I'd break up with him. I know that may sound a little extreme, but he's dismissing your feelings and refusing to work with you on a problem (and likely hiding something).

That said, I *really* don't think it'll get there. You two seemed to have a great relationship before all this, and I think you can have one after!

BEST. SEX. EVER.

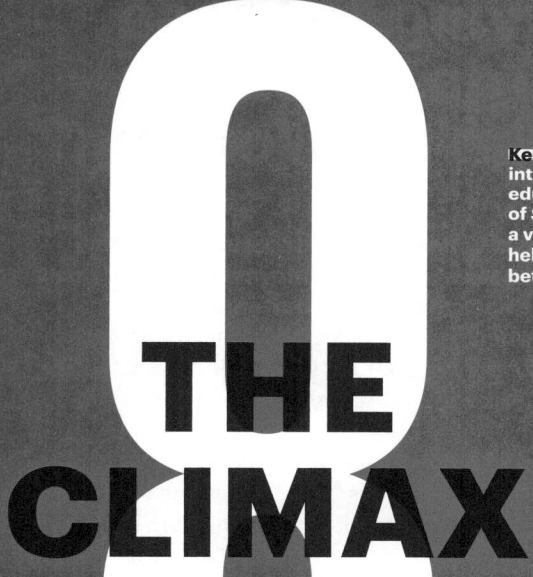

YOUR SEXPERT

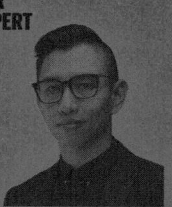

Kenneth Play is an international sex educator and the creator of *Sex Hacker Pro*, a video series for helping people become better lovers.

THE CLIMAX

It's the moment you've all been waiting for. Find out everything to know about orgasms— in all their delicious varieties.

CHAPTER 8

THE CLIMAX

I'm Trying to Close the Orgasm Gap. Why Isn't It Working?

You're a sex hacker, meaning you experiment to help people find the easiest ways to achieve their sexual goals. So...can people hack their way to better orgasms?
PLAY: Usually when people struggle with sexuality early on, they feel like they're doomed for life. But orgasm, like any other skill, is a trainable thing.

So how does orgasm hacking work, exactly?
There are three factors. One is: Are you getting the tactile sensation or stimulation that you need in order for your unique brain and body to have an orgasm? The second thing is: Are you having the right context that arouses you? Sex is such a contextual thing. Like, to have your butthole touched by a doctor examining you is very different than a lover touching your butthole; it's the exact same touch, but the context really dictates the experience. The third part is about mindfulness. Are you paying enough attention and connecting with your partner that you're experiencing it fully?

Once you get good at orgasm, it gets easier; there's a compound interest—just like the more fit you get, the easier it is to work out.

What about giving someone else an orgasm? Everyone's body is different and everyone's desires are different, but you teach certain universal rules for how to make someone cum. What are they?
You have to learn how to feel first—like paying attention to erotic cues. Then you have to learn how to calibrate—like how to touch until you find that it's effective. Then

you have to connect with them in a way that you can synchronize and flow—like you're dancing with a partner. And *then* you can add your moves, because if you feel like you're just following along, it's not fun. You have to express yourself. If you follow these stages, it really works.

A lot of well-intentioned guys are so focused on giving orgasms, they end up pressuring their partners and actually decreasing the likelihood of climax. What's your advice to those men?

There are so many other motivations for people to have sex beyond just orgasm, although I don't want to diminish the importance of orgasm at the same time. I think what people struggle with is performance anxiety. Say, in a hetero couple situation: The guy [thinks], *If I can make her cum, then I'm worthy as a man.* And then *she* feels a bunch of performance anxiety. She cannot get aroused if she's not feeling relaxed and safe.

We know that being pressured to orgasm is not going to lead to a better experience. I think better communication all around will bring the best out of that situation.

Say What Now?

What's *Anorgasmia*?

Anorgasmia—also known as Coughlan's syndrome—is the scientific term for when a person can't have an orgasm, despite sexual stimulation. There's *primary anorgasmia*, when a person has never been able to orgasm in their life, and *secondary anorgasmia*, when a person loses the ability to orgasm. There are many possible psychological and physiological causes of anorgasmia, so the best first step is talking to your doctor about what you're experiencing.

THE CLIMAX

What Is an Orgasm, Anyway?

So the funny thing is, scientists are still trying to figure it out. The challenge is that orgasms vary from person to person. They can come from stimulating the penis, clitoris, prostate, anus, nipples…heck, some folks can even think themselves to orgasm. "It's very hard to universally say, 'This will feel like *this* and *that*,'" Play says. "But there are some patterns that most people fall into."

What scientists *can* agree on: An orgasm represents a pleasurable peak in a sexual experience, dividing the buildup of tension from the release of tension. (Sex researchers William H. Master and Virginia E. Johnson described the journey in four phases: excitement, plateau, orgasm, and resolution.) "That's a universal biology thing: We get hungry, and we get satisfied," Play says. "I think that's the best answer we have right now."

BEST. SEX. EVER.

Can People With a Penis Have Multiple Orgasms?

If you have a penis, then you're probably used to feeling tapped out after climaxing. You can thank what's known as the *refractory period*—i.e., the period of time immediately following ejaculation when the brain becomes unresponsive to sexual stimulation. (The length of time varies from person to person; it could be anywhere from a few minutes to a day.)

Unless your junk is a scientific miracle, you won't have much luck achieving multiple ejaculatory orgasms without a refractory period in between. However, with a lot of practice, you might be able to have multiple non-ejaculatory orgasms. "It just requires a lot of training to separate ejaculation from the objective experience of orgasm," Play says.

When you're masturbating, try squeezing your pubococcygeal muscle (it should feel like stopping a pee midstream) to prevent yourself from releasing semen right at the brink of ejaculation. You may know this technique as edging. Work at it over time, paying close attention to the sensations in your body, and you may find you're able to separate the experiences of ejaculation and orgasm. We know it sounds corny, but the key here is allowing yourself to *feel your feelings*. "If you allow yourself to feel, those sensations will become more available to you because you'll know how to focus on them," Play says. You'll be in the right headspace to have all *kinds* of new orgasms.

THE CLIMAX

Does That Include Prostate Orgasms?

Heck yes. In fact, if you ask Play, the best way to achieve multiple orgasms involves having a prostate orgasm, a unique and satisfying sensation that doesn't necessarily involve penile ejaculation. Some penis-owners can have a prostate orgasm without even being hard, and the recovery time is a lot faster, Play says from personal experience and anecdotes from many others.

Some people compare a penile orgasm to an external clitoral orgasm and a prostate orgasm to an internal G-spot orgasm; in other words, they say the P-spot orgasm is more of a full-body experience than a penile orgasm.

When working toward a P-spot climax, most people will start by stimulating the penis and prostate together. "The penis is like the high scorer that keeps the morale up, and then you bring in the prostate and you're like, 'Holy shit! I didn't know the prostate could assist!'" Play says. "Then you realize the prostate can do it by itself."

The following section is Play's step-by-step guide for achieving multiple orgasms through prostate stimulation.

Start with masturbation.

"First of all, I recommend masturbation rather than partner play to start this exploration because you have a direct feedback loop, and without having to instruct someone else or worry about being comfortable, things are much simpler and more effective," Play says. "Put on your favorite porn or whatever you normally do to get in the mood. Start stimulating your penis to get to a certain level of arousal before anal penetration, because otherwise it can feel like a medical exam."

Use a prostate toy to help you reach the P-spot. (See page 108 for the different types of butt-friendly toys available!)

"Move the toy around until you find the right spot, then use a rocking motion with your wrist joint to rock the [toy] against the front wall of the rectum, applying pressure to the prostate," Play says.

Combine prostate stimulation with your regular masturbation routine.

"Start playing with the toy until you feel some sensation on your prostate," Play says. "As you get close to orgasm, the prostate stimulation will start to feel way better than you ever thought it could. The first goal is just to have a blended orgasm while stimulating your prostate.

"Next time, do the same technique but direct your attention even more to the sensations that are coming from your penis. Use stimulation of the penis to increase arousal, but as you get closer to orgasm, decrease or stop stimulating your penis and keep stimulating your prostate."

Bask in the (refractory-period-free) wonders of the prostate orgasm.

"Keep trying to edge yourself to orgasm, but stop stimulating your penis and try to get your prostate to be the one to push you over the hump," Play says. "Instead of tensing, relax deeply and focus on your prostate and the sensations from stimulation. Do this enough that it gets you [to the climax]. Once you do, you'll learn a completely different type of orgasm. It feels more like a full-body orgasm and is very different than the kind you've had from penile stimulation.

"The more you do this, the more prostate stimulation you can apply, the more prostate orgasms you can have. To my surprise, what I've found is that after I have a prostate orgasm, my penis stays hard and is still responsive to sexual stimulation. If you continue to masturbate by touching your penis, you can immediately have another orgasm."

THE CLIMAX

Can You Tell Me More About Multiple Penile Orgasms?

It's possible as Play mentioned earlier, but it requires a ton of practice to be able to orgasm without releasing any semen (and in turn, triggering the refractory period). The technique of climaxing multiple times sans ejaculation is known as non-ejaculatory multiple orgasm, or NEMO.

"Taoist traditions have extremely elaborate methods for cultivating this ability, as well as some yogic lineages from India, Tibet, and China," Play explains. "These traditions use this practice to retain energy and alertness and direct it toward the goals of their tradition."

The key to NEMO is learning how to identify the point at which ejaculation feels inevitable, then contracting your pelvic-floor muscles to stop it from happening as you orgasm. Doing Kegels in your spare time—hell, do 'em while you read this book!—will give you maximum control over those muscles. Deep belly breathing can also help you delay ejaculation as you focus on the feelings of pleasure. The resulting non-ejaculatory orgasm will feel smaller than your usual climax, but on the bright side, you can keep on doin' it.

BEST. SEX. EVER.

CONFESSIONS

"The Difference Between Prostate and Penile Orgasms Is…"

"Almost going blind with pleasure (prostate orgasms) and a form of indifference along the lines of *Oh, I came* (penile orgasms)." **—Slade, 32**

"Prostate orgasms are whole-body experiences for me. They feel 'thorough' or 'complete.' Often, if I just get off without that stimulation, it feels like it's more on the 'surface' level. It's similar to the way my wife describes the difference between orgasms that stem from external clitoral stimulation versus those that come from G-spot stimulation." **—Ben, 43**

"Prostate orgasms are deeper. It's like they originate in your body instead of your dick. I have to catch my breath afterward, and my whole body is shaking from the tension that slowly builds up and then gets released in an explosion." **—Curtis, 38**

"No comparison. The penile orgasm is concentrated, protracted, and short. On the other hand, you have prostate orgasms, which seem to build more, come in waves, and wash over the whole body repeatedly." **—Alex, 30**

"A prostate orgasm is so spiritual, and a penile orgasm is a bit more mechanical—but still incredible." **—George, 29**

What's the Best Way for a Person With a Vulva to Reach Orgasm?

As you'll recall from the beginning of the chapter, everyone climaxes differently. Despite what you may have heard, there's no magic trick that can make *anyone* with a vulva reach orgasm.

That said, research has shown that the majority of people with a vulva can't orgasm from penetration alone. An oft-cited 2017 paper in the *Journal of Sex & Marital Therapy* found that 36.6 percent of vulva-owners also require external clitoral stimulation; a further 36 percent said they don't *need* that clit stimulation but it sure does improve the experience. Just 18.4 percent of respondents said they were happy with vaginal penetration on its own, and yet—as Play points out—there's still this stigma that if a vulva-owner can't cum from internal stimulation alone, there's something wrong with them.

"The clitoris is no different than the head of your penis, as far as the nerve that stimulates your brain," he says. Expecting a vulva-owner to orgasm from internal stimulation alone would be like telling a penis-owner: "You have to orgasm from me penetrating your butt with a dildo, and if you don't cum, there's something wrong with you!"

BEST. SEX. EVER.

What's the G-Spot? (And Does It Exist?)

Named after Ernst Gräfenberg, the German researcher who first identified it in the 1940s, the G-spot has long been portrayed—inaccurately—as a mythical pleasure button hidden on the anterior (front) wall of the vagina.

Researchers have since determined that the G-spot isn't some independent, mystical entity; instead, it's an erogenous zone linked partly to the clitoris, which extends up to five inches inside the body. A major 2014 paper in *Nature Reviews* came to the following conclusion: "The anatomical relationships and dynamic interactions between the clitoris, urethra, and anterior vaginal wall have led to the concept of a clitourethrovaginal (CUV) complex…that, when properly stimulated during penetration, could induce orgasmic responses."

But hey, we get it: "G-spot" is a whole lot easier to say than "clitourethrovaginal complex." The main takeaway here is that some people enjoy stimulating the front wall of the vagina. It's one of about a billion things you can do during sex, so don't worry if it's not your or your partner's thing.

Pro Tip: ➡ It's All About the Blend

Blended orgasm is a term used to describe an orgasm that comes from external clitoral stimulation combined with stimulation from one or more other erogenous zones, such as the G-spot, anus, cervix, and nipples. (Think a person with a vulva climaxing from holding a vibrator on their clitoris during penetration—and wearing nipple clamps and/or a butt plug at the same time.)

THE CLIMAX

THE BEST POSITIONS FOR...
VULVA-OWNERS TO CLIMAX

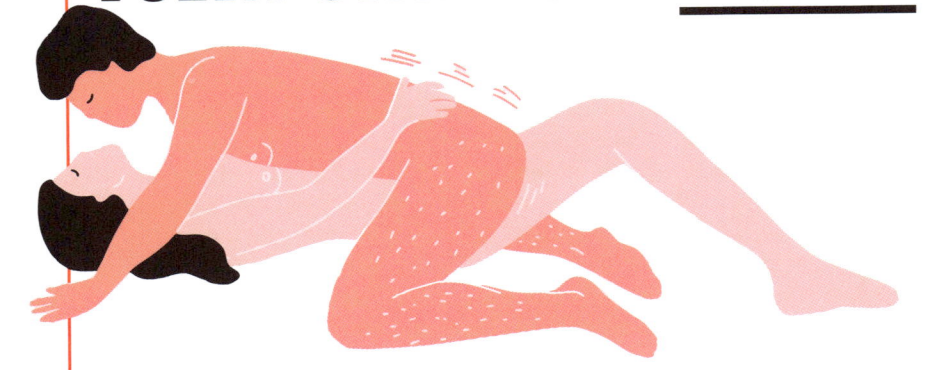

↑ MISSIONARY WITH A VIBRATING COCK RING

It's the same as classic missionary (see page 62), but the penetrating partner wears a vibrating cock ring to stimulate the receiver's clit.

↓ THE BUTTERFLY

This position tilts the vulva-owner's pelvis to a prime angle for G-spot stimulation. Plus, it gives the penetrating partner plenty of space to put their fingers (or a vibrator) to good use.

↓ COITAL ALIGNMENT TECHNIQUE (CAT)

In this position, the partner with a vulva should lie on their back with their legs spread comfortably, as they would in missionary position. On top of them, the person doing the penetrating should raise themselves on their arms with their shoulders high and their back arched. The key is for the penetrating partner to shift forward, so their penis or dildo is pressed against their partner's pelvis pointing down rather than up. This way, they rub against their partner's external clitoris on their way to entering the vagina.

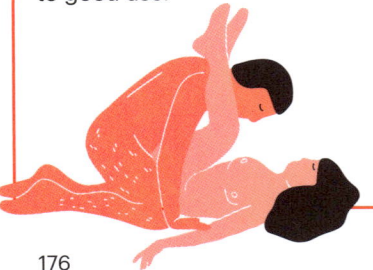

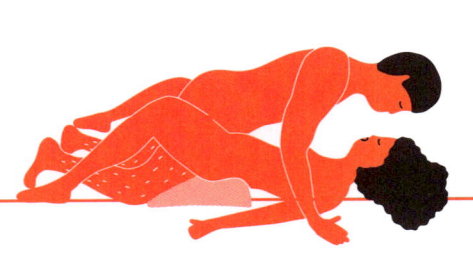

BEST. SEX. EVER.

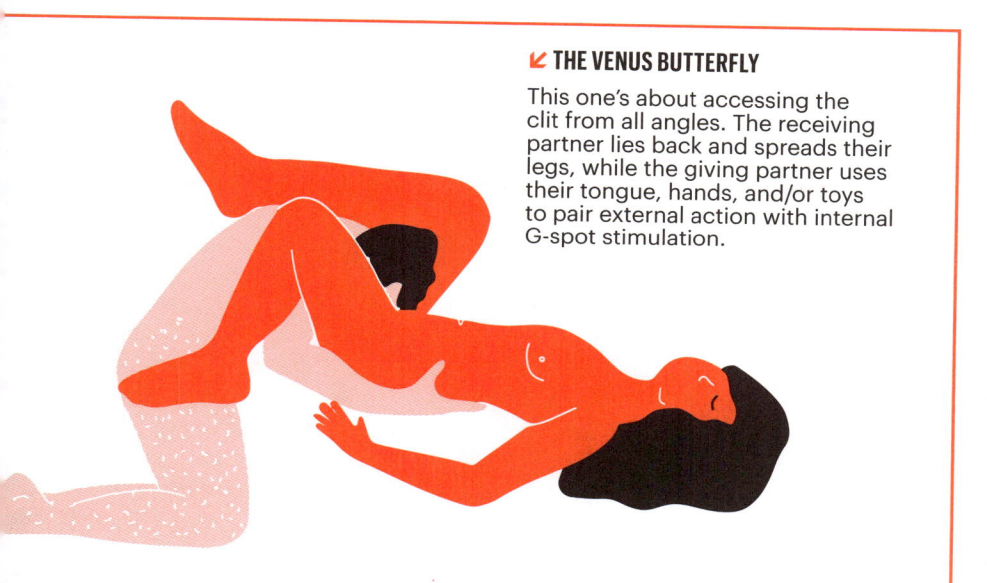

↙ THE VENUS BUTTERFLY

This one's about accessing the clit from all angles. The receiving partner lies back and spreads their legs, while the giving partner uses their tongue, hands, and/or toys to pair external action with internal G-spot stimulation.

Say What Now?

What's *Squirting*?

When some people with a vulva have an orgasm, they're able to "squirt" a clear-ish liquid through their urethra—kinda like how people with a penis are able to ejaculate, except in this case, the process has nothing to do with reproduction. A 2011 paper published in *The Journal of Sexual Medicine* found that most people's squirt is watered-down urine, sometimes including a *tiiiiny* bit of female ejaculate: a white, milklike substance produced in the Skene's glands.

Vulva-owners can orgasm without squirting—so why the cultural fascination with this random sex act? According to Play, it's that our brain seeks visual and auditory confirmation that we've done something correctly. "Female ejaculation does not equal orgasm, but we crave the sign-off," he says.

THE CLIMAX

SEXPLAIN IT

Dear Sexplain It,

I'm a 30-year-old gay man, and no one can make me orgasm. Only I can do it, when I'm masturbating alone. I can't orgasm from bottoming and especially not from topping. I can't even cum from handjobs. I'm sure it's psychological. I just don't even know how to start addressing this issue without speaking to a therapist. But even finding the right one to deal with something like this is a daunting task in itself.

—Needs Release

BEST. SEX. EVER.

Dear Needs Release,

I think you're dealing with performance anxiety. If you also had trouble orgasming by yourself, I'd say it might be a physical problem. But since you have no problem climaxing solo, it sounds like it's all psychological, as you suggested.

It's an unfortunate reality that some of our first sexual experiences can set the tone for the rest of our sex life. I was so goddamn nervous the first time I attempted to have sex with my girlfriend that I couldn't get erect. This led to years of on-and-off erectile dysfunction. It was awful. But I eventually learned to break the cycle with some help from a therapist and friends.

To break your own cycle of anorgasmia, you're going to have to remove all this pressure you've placed on yourself to orgasm and be more present in the sexual experience. I know this is significantly easier said than done, and "chill out," on its own, is god-awful advice. That's why I want to give you multiple actionable items to help you relax.

Item 1: Let your partners know that you have trouble orgasming during sex. I was able to start getting erect when I told my sex partners beforehand: "Hey, just to let you know, I sometimes can't get hard, especially when I'm crushing on someone. If I don't get hard, it's not because I don't find you attractive. I'm just a little nervous." Most loved hearing that, and they'd tell me not to worry. Then, do you know what happened when I knew it was totally okay if I couldn't get hard? I GOT HARD.

Item 2: Let's remove orgasming from the pedestal you've placed it on. "An orgasm isn't the be-all and end-all of a gratifying sexual experience," says sex columnist and educator Bobby Box. "When you're anxious about having an orgasm while having sex, you're removed from enjoying the experience." I know that in every gay porno ever, the bottom shoots on his abs as he gets plowed on his back, but that's not happening every single time we run-of-the-mill non-porn-stars bone. I can't even stay *hard* when I'm on the receiving end of a dick or strap-on—it's simply too much intensity for me. That doesn't mean I'm not enjoying the sexual experience.

Item 3: Try mutual masturbation with your partners, which will help you get used to finishing in the presence of someone else. (I know that in itself can be anxiety-inducing!) Once you get that down, you might find it easier to orgasm when you're touching one another.

Last but not least, item 4: See a therapist. I know it takes a lot of effort to find someone who is affordable, has availability, and is adept at dealing with LGBTQ+ specific issues, but it's worth putting in the work. Psychology Today (psychologytoday.com) is a nationwide resource you can use; it has filters, so you can search for a therapist who works explicitly with gay men.

In the meantime, cut yourself some slack. You may be surprised to find that in doing so, you get that sweet, sweet release you so desperately crave.

BEST. SEX. EVER.

YOUR SEXPERT

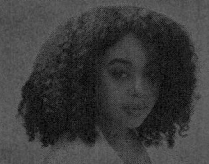

Shadeen Francis is a licensed marriage and family therapist specializing in sex therapy, emotional intelligence, and social justice.

CHAPTER 9
CLOSING LINES

Sex doesn't finish the moment you do. From cleanup to cuddling, learn what to do after the act to make the next time even better.

CLOSING LINES

How Do I Tell Them the Sex Could Have Been Better?

"Did you cum?" isn't the greatest question to ask a partner when you're done having sex. Can you talk about why?
FRANCIS: I want that question to come earlier. If [couples are] having conversations about sex *before* they start having sex, that would be an ideal time to ask questions about pleasure and orgasm: "What makes you feel good? What will I see and hear when you are enjoying yourself? I want to really, really make sure that you're having a good time." Being able to have that questioning beforehand saves us a lot of grief in the long run and improves the quality of our connections during [sex].

If you want to tell a partner what did or didn't work for you during a hookup—call it a "postgame analysis"—when's the best time to bring that up?
It's going to depend very much on style. Some folks like the immediate replay and consider it sexy postcoital pillow talk. Some folks are still overstimulated or sleepy. It'll be up to the people involved to determine when might be a good time. That's something that ideally can be negotiated.

How can you signal to your partner that you'd like to have that talk?
"You know, I'd love to talk about last night. What was really good for you? What would you like more of for next time? What would you like to be different next time?" And [it's important] to be able to name some of the context for this conversation, like "It feels really important to me for us to have a sex life that feels really good to both of us."

What would you say to someone who gave their partner honest feedback about something that didn't work and the partner was really offended?
We are ultimately looking for partners who prioritize our pleasure above their ego. However, we also live in a culture that positions sex as some form of character trait. While sex is behavioral, somehow we've come into this narration of sex that it literally says something about you as a person. For me to name what I like on my body is actually not a critique or criticism of anybody else. What we're encountering there is a sex education gap that we might be able to bridge if we have the energy and interest in doing so—to be able to [say to] this person, "This feedback isn't actually a criticism of you. This is me telling you what feels good on my body. I'm telling you this because I want us to continue. I want us to have good experiences with each other. And so I want you to know what feels good to me."

Let's say you had a really great first date or first hookup with a new partner and you want to see them again. There's a lot of conflicting information out there about how soon you should let them know. What do you recommend?
I think we've really come to overcomplicate so much of this. We are simple creatures living complicated lives. For what [technology] has done to increase the possibilities of connection, I think that we've also used technology in a way that has somehow made connection feel more confusing. We've reached a place where we've vilified vulnerability as [being] weak. I think it's an important part of being human and having pleasurable experiences: We have to open ourselves up to the risk of being impacted positively—and sometimes not so positively. So, that's a long preamble to the answer of: *Literally just tell them.* If you want something, say it.

CLOSING LINES

Why Is the Post-Sex Cleanup So Awkward?

In movie sex scenes, couples always seem to pump their way to a spectacular simultaneous climax, slump over, turn off the bedside lamps, and fall asleep. This cinematic routine is infuriating, and not just because it sets unrealistic expectations about how easy it is for everyone to orgasm—particularly people with a vulva. It also completely ignores the inevitable post-sex cleanup! Do they *really* expect us to believe that no one has to shower, throw out a used condom, or pee?

Perhaps it's often excluded because the post-sex cleanup can feel awkward and unromantic. (If you've ever waddled to the bathroom with a handful of bodily fluid, you probably know what we mean.) But it doesn't have to be that way—not if you view the cleanup as a natural extension of the sex session. "It doesn't actually have to be a break from this affectionate, erotic, or intimate energy," Francis says. "Maybe we both get up and go to the bathroom. Maybe we both take a shower. Maybe we clean each other off."

Pro Tip: ➡ Prep Your Bed for Action

Sex is way more fun and freeing when you don't have to stress about staining the sheets. That's why we recommend investing in a waterproof blanket or bedsheet. (Google "waterproof sex blanket" or "waterproof sex sheet," and you should find plenty of options.) Go forth and drizzle that lube with reckless abandon.

BEST. SEX. EVER.

To make the transition as smooth as possible, plan ahead. Before you get going, leave a bottle of water and paper towels or a microfiber cloth next to the bed. If you know you like having some alone time to clean up, you can mention it to your partner beforehand too. When it comes time to pop to the bathroom, keep it casual and tell them you'll BRB. "We can continue that playful, sexual, erotic, and affectionate energy while doing something that is really normal, which is taking care of our bodies," Francis says.

Pro Tip: ➡ Properly Clean Your Most Prized Possessions

Whatever parts you have, peeing after sex helps to flush away bacteria and prevent urinary tract infections, or UTIs. When it comes to rinsing off, opt for gentle soap and warm water—no fancy wet wipes or other "spring rain"–scented cleansing products necessary.

And don't forget to clean your sex toys after each use to prevent skin and yeast infections. Soap and water will typically do the trick, but you should double-check each toy's cleaning guide for any further washing and drying directions.

CLOSING LINES

What Is Sexual Aftercare?

Sex is an *experience*. Whether you're vanilla AF or all about the kinky stuff we covered in Chapter 6, getting it on can leave you physically, mentally, and emotionally spent. Just like you'd stretch your sore muscles or collapse on the couch after a punishing workout, engaging in the ritual known as sexual aftercare can help you wind down after an intense romp.

"Aftercare is a way in which we maintain connection to people after 'play,'" Francis says—*play* meaning any kind of sexy activity. "It's the things you do to make sure that everyone at the end of this sexual experience...is safe enough or feeling taken care of enough."

Everyone's needs are different, so aftercare routines will vary between partners and sex sessions. Maybe it's cuddling or eating snacks or watching something funny on TV. If you dabble in BDSM, which often involves immersive role play, you might choose a ritual that helps guide you back to reality; if you're submissive—for example—and you've just been humiliated by a dominant partner, you might want your partner to hold you close and whisper all the things they love about you. "There's any number of things folks might need," Francis says, and it's important for partners to communicate those needs to each other.

Here are a few more examples of the endless ways to practice sexual aftercare:

- Taking a shower or bath together
- Trading massages
- Rubbing soothing balm onto sore body parts
- Passing a partner their mobility device (e.g., a cane or crutch) to get out of bed
- Rehydrating with water (or hot herbal tea for added relaxation)
- Recounting the experience that you just had (and highlighting what you liked about it)
- Gently kissing or making out
- Falling asleep in each other's arms
- Cleaning up the room
- Giving each other alone time
- Planning a romantic date with your primary partner following a group sex experience

Pro Tip: ➡ Aftercare Extends to the Next Day Too

The *after* in aftercare doesn't just apply to the moments immediately following your sex session. Making a partner feel loved and supported can also mean texting them the next day to thank them for a fun experience and see how they're doing.

CLOSING LINES

CONFESSIONS

"My Favorite Form of Aftercare Is…"

"Food and cuddles. I love to get intimate after sex and enjoy the afterglow of an orgasm and swap sweat. It's nice to recap the events of the night and talk about it sweetly. I'm also almost always starving after a long fuck session, so finding the nearest burger joint is so satisfying. (I kinda need the food after a bottoming diet.)"
—Tim, 28 (See page 102 for more details on that diet.)

"A few minutes of just lying there and catching my breath, then a slow transition to cuddling. Usually pretty low on talking for a bit, since it's nice to just soak in the serenity of the situation. Once conversation gets going again, some affectionate, flirtatious humor mixed with making out makes my cold, dead heart flutter."
—David, 29

"I prefer to meditate and sit with the feelings of expenditure. Particularly following a long anal sex session, I love the feeling of being used up." **—Edward, 52**

"A warm, wet washcloth and some snuggling nekkid. It's just a great way to feel connected to the person you were with." **—Nate, 43**

"Lots of cuddling and kindness. I love it anyway, and it feels good to be supportive, especially after doing terrible things to a willing participant." **—Matthew, 35**

BEST. SEX. EVER.

Why Does Cuddling Feel So Good?

It's science, baby—specifically, brain chemistry. When you hug or snuggle with a partner, your pituitary gland releases a chemical called oxytocin, which has been shown to reduce stress and promote bonding in relationships. (There's a reason oxytocin has been nicknamed the "love hormone"!) Other feel-good chemicals released during cuddling include dopamine, a neurotransmitter that helps you feel pleasure, and serotonin, a hormone that helps stabilize your mood.

In what sounds like a positively delightful area of research, scientists have linked cuddling to a number of mental, physical, and relationship benefits. A 2018 study published in the journal *PLOS One* found that people who received hugs were better able to handle interpersonal conflicts; another 2018 study published in the journal *PNAS* found a connection between hand-holding with a romantic partner and physical pain relief.

Just remember, not *everyone* wants to cuddle or to cuddle for the same amount of time. Ask your partner what feels good for them—and be specific, Francis says: "Is it just a five-minute cuddle and then I can roll over or get up, or are you the sort of person that wants a good half-hour snuggle fest?"

CLOSING LINES

THE BEST POSITIONS FOR...
CUDDLING

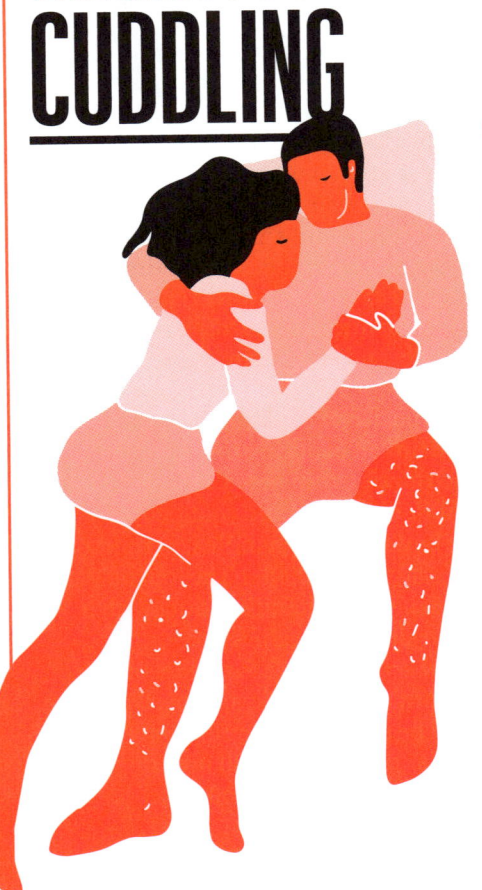

↙ HALF SPOON

Spooning can get a little steamy—in, like, a sweaty way. Especially if you've just had an energetic romp. Try this intimate variation to get a little more airflow between your bods.

HORIZONTAL HUG ↗

Lie on your sides, face-to-face, and wrap your arms and legs around each other. This one's great for kissing, gazing into each other's eyes, and basking in the glow of each other's satisfied smiles.

BEST. SEX. EVER.

THE LAP NAP ↘

One partner snuggles up between the other's legs and leans against their chest. Pro tip for the person in back: You're perfectly positioned to give a neck and shoulder massage.

THE BABY MONKEY ↘

Ever seen how a baby monkey rides around on its mom's back? It looks cozy as hell—hence this cuddling position. Close your eyes and you might just drift off to sleep.

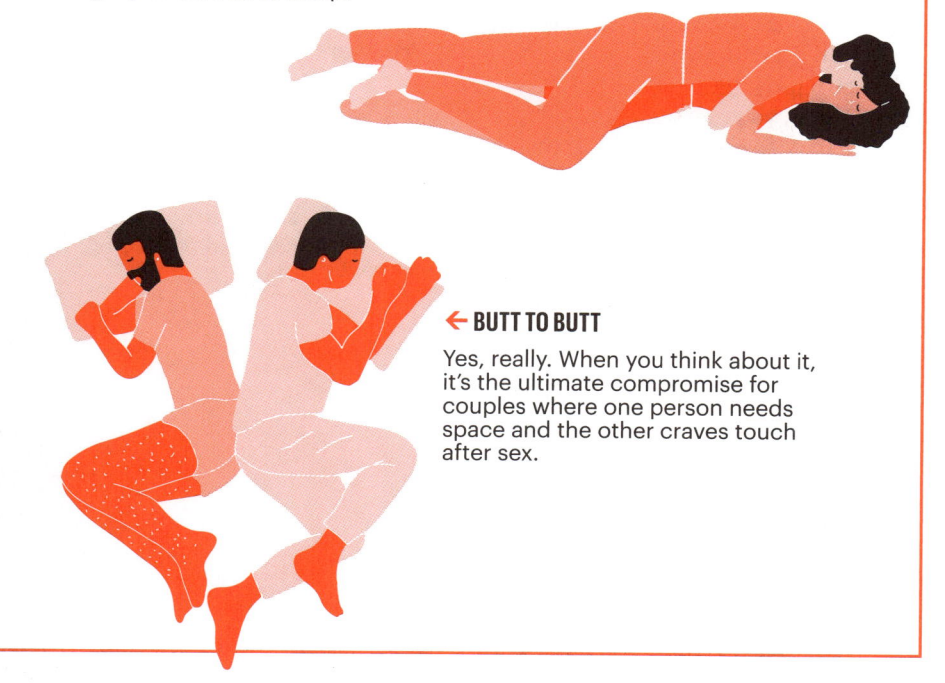

← BUTT TO BUTT

Yes, really. When you think about it, it's the ultimate compromise for couples where one person needs space and the other craves touch after sex.

CLOSING LINES

How Do I Tell a Partner I'd Like to Have Sex Again?

If you're in a relationship, we'll go ahead and assume your partner knows you're open to having sex with them again. But if you just hooked up with someone new, communicating your eagerness to do it again can feel a little more daunting. And we get it: There's a lot of mixed messaging out there about when and how to message someone after a good first encounter. Should you wait a few days so you don't seem desperate? Should you not message them at all and wait for them to message *you*?

Actually, it's option C: Embrace your vulnerable side and tell them how you feel—as soon as you're ready to share it (see page 183).

When you message them, don't make it a demand ("We have to do that again"). Instead, Francis recommends an open-ended message like this: "Hey! I had a really good time and I'd love to see you again, if you're open to it." If they turn you down, don't sweat it. You want—and deserve!—a partner who shares an enthusiastic desire to see you again.

THE BEST _____ EVER

The Best Text I've Ever Received After a First Date (or Hookup)

"My wife and I dated in high school, then broke up and married other people we met in college. We reconnected after we had both been divorced from our first spouses. We had an amazing (second) first date and ended up making out like high school kids in the parking lot of a bar we had drinks in after a movie. Afterward, she texted me and asked, 'Where the hell was that in high school?' Made my week." —**Nate, 43**

"'No guy has ever made me cum like that before—I've literally never cum twice in one session. I would like to see you again.'" —**Tim, 28**

"'Your smile is contagious. You completely rocked my world last night.'" —**Natalie, 37**

"A picture of the hickey I gave her." —**Christi, 24**

"That was the best and biggest I've ever had. So sore but will be back for more.'" —**Michael, 37**

CLOSING LINES

SEXPLAIN IT

(a) ——————————————▶ **(b)**

Dear Sexplain It,

My girlfriend is a badass type A boss who's good at telling people what to do. It's one of the things I find most attractive about her. The only time it sucks is after sex, when she's quick to tell me all the things I could have done differently. On the one hand, I want to know when I'm not doing a good job in bed and what things I could improve on. On the other hand, it makes me feel like I'm being scolded! How can we fix this dynamic? I want to be the best lover possible but am sick of feeling like a kid who just brought home a bad report card.

—**Bad Student**

Dear Bad Student,

It sounds like your girlfriend runs a tech start-up or a Fortune 500 company. I bet all day she's telling people what to do and her direct form of communication is how she successfully manages her team. But the thing is, you're not her employee. You're her boyfriend, who did not agree to any boss-employee sexual role play. It's perfectly fair to want sex without the scolding afterward, even if you also want to be as good a lover as possible. These two things are not mutually exclusive.

Before we get any further, I must ask: Is she critiquing the same things every time? If so, my advice is to listen to her—especially given everything we know about the orgasm gap. (Read more about the gendered disparity in orgasm frequency on page 66.) However, if she's constantly lobbing new critiques because that's just how she is, please continue reading.

Your girlfriend needs to learn how to turn off work mode the moment you two are together. She also may not realize she's doing it unless you tell her. Lucky for you, she seems well versed in direct and honest communication, so as long as she can dish it *and* take it, I think this convo shouldn't be *too* difficult.

I showed your question to Kate Balestrieri, Psy.D., founder of the therapy center Modern Intimacy, and she agreed that "direct and assertive" communication is your best approach. "Let your girlfriend know the effect her delivery has on you and offer different ways her feedback could be more impactful," Balestrieri says.

At a time when you're not about to have sex (or you didn't just finish having it), tell your partner that you have something you'd like to bring up with

CLOSING LINES

her. Say, "I love having sex with you, but receiving negative feedback *immediately* after sex doesn't make me feel good." (BTW, it's one of the worst types of aftercare imaginable. You probably want to cuddle, and meanwhile, she's pointing out all your flaws.) Then continue, "I'm all for sharing how we felt about our last hookup, but I'd like for it to happen a little farther out from the act—and for it to be more of a two-way conversation."

From there, establish a new plan for how the two of you can share what you *both* want more of in the bedroom. I feel like your girlfriend loves planning meetings—she'd probably be down for a standing Wednesday-night sex talk on the couch. However you decide to schedule this, "you can give each other feedback on what works and what isn't quite striking a chord," Balestrieri says.

Deploying this plan will save you from getting scolded immediately after sex, but I also want to give you tools for if she uses your new debriefs to unfairly berate you. If you feel like you just can't do *anything* right, say something like, "It would be more helpful if you could tell me exactly what it is you want me to do and when." At this point, you'll have given her the fullest opportunity to express what she wants, and—I assume—you'll have responded to the best of your ability in the bedroom. If she's still criticizing you the same way after that, you have more of a leg to stand on when you tell her you don't appreciate her behavior. And if she's not willing to compromise, well, it's up to you whether this is the person you want to be with long-term.

Also, feel free to tell her what *she* can do better in bed. I'm sure there's something else you'd like that hasn't come up yet. Get creative. Maybe *you* get to be dominant in bed. That'll give her a nice break from always being the boss.

BEST. SEX. EVER.

i

INDEX

INDEX

A

after sex, 181–196
    aftercare guidelines and tips, 186–187
    best texts received after first date/hookup, 193
    cleanup tips, 184–185
    cuddling appeal, 189
    cuddling positions, 190–191
    favorite forms of aftercare, 188
    the next day, 187
    Sexplain It column (Bad Student), 194–196
    telling partner you'd like to have sex again, 192
    telling them sex could have been better, 182–183
alcohol, ED and, 77, 80
amount of sex
    excessive masturbation, 158
    getting back to more sex, 23
    honeymoon phase and, 24
    mismatched desire patterns and, 24–25
    non-sex issues influencing, 25
anal beads, 67, 109, 116
anal play/sex, 95–118
    bottoming, 101
    classic DP (double penetration) position, 138
    cleaning out your butt, 103–104
    condoms and, 59, 159–160
    confessions, 22, 100–101
    doggy style position, 63
    eating the booty (anilingus), 110–113
    fingering techniques, 106–107
    getting over stigma of, 96–97
    lube for, 60–61, 99, 106–107, 160
    poop and, 102–105
    porn myths, 160
    prepping for, 103–107
    sex toys and, 67, 69 (See also anal beads; butt plugs; dildos; prostate massagers)
    Sexplain It column (Obsessed With Anal), 116–118
    topping, 100
    train position (daisy chain) and, 139
    training kits, 109
    warm-up techniques, 106–107
    why people love it, 99–101
anal toys, 108–109. See also anal beads; butt plugs; dildos; prostate massagers
anilingus 69 position, 113
anorgasmia, 167, 179
asking for sex. See consent, asking for sex
authors, backgrounds and this book, 11

B

baby monkey position, 191
balls, involving, 51, 150
BDSM, 120–122, 123, 125, 143–144
best sex ever
    about
        authors' backgrounds and, 11
        this book and, 6, 9–12
    envisioning yours, 9
    oral sex testimonials, 56
    positions for (See positions, categories of; positions, specific)
    texts received after first date/hookup, 193
    threesome/group sex testimonials, 135
bisexuals, 30, 99, 135, 139
blended orgasm, 175

BEST. SEX. EVER.

blood pressure, ED and, 79
blowjobs
    best positions for, 54–55
    bringing balls into, 51
    doggy blowjob position, 139
    Sexplain It column (Just Wants Head), 70–72
    upping your game, 50–51
bodily fluids fantasies, 124
Brahmbhatt, Jamin, about, 73
butt plugs, 42, 67, 69, 104, 108–109, 118
butt to butt position, 191
butterfly position, 176

C

captain position, 114
Caraballo, Jor-El, about, 13
classic DP (double penetration) position, 138
cleaning up after sex, 184–185
climax. *See* ejaculation; orgasms
clitoris
    blended orgasm and, 175
    coital alignment technique (CAT) and, 176
    cowgirl position and, 62
    dirty talk and, 43
    G-spot and, 175
    happy baby pose and, 115
    masturbation and, 154
    missionary position with vibrating cock ring and, 176
    oral sex positions, 52–53
    outercourse and, 49
    pretzel position and, 89
    reaching orgasm and, 174–175
    sex toys and, 66–67, 69, 94, 150
    upping your oral game, 50–51
    Venus butterfly position and, 177
closed for business position, 53
cock rings, 68, 85, 157
cock rings, vibrating, 67, 157, 176
coital alignment technique (CAT), 176
communication. *See also* dirty talk; sexting
    about kinks and fetishes, 126–127
    feedback on performance, 182–183, 194–196
    getting back to more sex and, 23
    getting verbal, 128
    importance of, 7
    post-sex (*See* after sex)
    telling partner what you like, 7
condoms
    best, types and characteristics, 57–58
    porn myths, 159–160
    pros and cons, 57–59
    wearing, 59
confessions
    "My favorite form of aftercare is...," 188
    "My funniest first time was...," 22
    "My most awkward group sex experience was...," 142
    "The difference between prostate and penile orgasms is...," 173
    "The hottest sext I've ever received was...," 37
    "Why I love bottoming...," 101
    "Why I love topping...," 100
confidence, developing and projecting, 15
consent, asking for sex
    asking for enthusiastic consent, 17–18
    confidence in, 15

INDEX

enthusiastic consent, 16–18
flirty vs. creepy approaches, 14–15
if you're unsure, stop!, 18
language that affirms partner, 18
"no means no," 16
"yes means yes," 16
cowgirl
    cowgirl position, 62
    double cowgirl position, 136
    extended reverse cowgirl position, 115
    reverse cowgirl position, 65
    squatting cowgirl position, 115
cuckolding, 125
cuddling, appeal of, 189
cuddling, positions for, 190–191

D

diabetes, ED and, 79
dildos, 67, 69, 108–109
dirty talk, 31–46. *See also* photos, nude; sexting
    building your own (worksheet), 44
    degrading terms and, 32–33
    descriptive words for, 43
    fear of using, 32
    getting verbal, 128
    in #MeToo era, 32–33
    name calling, 128
    Sexplain It column (Failed Dirty Talker), 45–46
    sexting tips and confessions, 34–37
    what to say in bed, 42–44
doggy blowjob position, 139
doggy deluxe position, 137
doggy style position, 63, 112
doggy train position, 136
dominant roles, 54, 97, 120, 123, 127
double cowgirl position, 136
double oral position, 137
drink kiss, 21
drugs, ED and, 77

E

ED (erectile dysfunction). *See* performance
ED medications, 74, 78
edging, 82, 149–150, 169
Eiffel Tower/spit roast position, 138
ejaculation. See also orgasms
    female, squirting, 160, 177
    keep going after, 83
    lasting longer, 48, 81–83, 153 (*See also* edging)
    masturbation and, 153
    refractory period, 169, 171, 172
Engle, Gigi, about, 31
enthusiastic consent, 16–18
erections
    condoms and, 58
    ED and (*See* performance)
    masturbation optimizing, 153
    size of, 84–85, 92–93
    stronger, cock ring for, 68, 85, 157
exhibitionism, 124
extended reverse cowgirl position, 115
eye contact, kissing and, 21

F

face-off position, 64
face-sitter position (blowjob), 54
face-sitting position (anal), 113
fetishes. *See* kinks and fetishes
flat iron position, 27
foreplay. *See* blowjobs; kissing; oral sex; sex toys
Francis, Shadeen, about, 181

G

gay men, 30, 49, 99, 178, 180
gender play, 124–125
gift wrapped position, 26
group sex. *See* threesomes and group sex
G-spot
    about, 175
    anal stimulation and, 96
    blended orgasm and, 175
    positions to stimulate, 62, 176–177
    sex toys and, 67, 94
G-whiz position, 88

H

hacking, orgasm, 166
half spoon position, 190
happy baby pose, 115
heart disease, ED and, 79
heir to the throne position, 52
honeymoon phase, 24
horizontal hug position, 190
hot seat position, 64
Howard, Shamyra, about, 145
hump and blow position, 54
hypertension, ED and, 79

I

ice kiss, 21
impact play, 130
intercourse. *See also* positions, categories of; positions, specific
    balanced perspective on, 49
    classic positions, 62–63
    lasting longer, 48, 81–83
    lube for, 60–61
    outercourse and, 49
    procreation and, 48–49

J

jelqing, 87

K

Kegels, 81–82, 172
Kerner, Ian, about, 47
kinks and fetishes, 119–144. *See also* threesomes and group sex
    bringing into the bedroom, 128–130
    common fetishes, 120
    common kinks, 123–125
    definitions of, 120
    impact play, 130

INDEX

    menu/checklist of (yes/no/maybe), 131
    origins/development of, 121
    role play, 129
    safe word importance, 125
    Sexplain It column (Kinky in Florida), 143–144
    stigmas toward, 121–122
    switches (both dominant and submissive) and, 127
    talking with partner about, 126–127, 131
kissing
    biochemistry of attraction and, 19
    biting or sucking carefully, 20
    creative ideas, 21
    drink kiss and ice kiss, 21
    eye contact and, 21
    getting in sync with partner, 21
    hair and, 20
    mixing depth of kiss, 20
    moving slowly, 19
    partner's cues and, 19
    softening tongue and lips, 20
    tips for pro kissing, 19–21
    vampire kiss, 21
Kivin method, 53

L

lap nap position, 191
launchpad position, 90
legs on shoulders position, 115
Lehmiller, Justin, about, 119
locked and loaded position, 26
lube, 60–61, 99, 106–107, 153, 160
lying blow position, 55

M

masturbation, 145–164
    after workout, 158
    bringing balls into, 150
    edging and, 82, 149–150, 169
    excessive, 158
    fighting premature ejaculation with, 82–83
    health benefits of, 152–153
    how to step up your game, 146–147
    lubes to use in a pinch, 153
    multiple penis orgasms and, 169–172
    mutual, 154–155, 180
    new ways to experience, 148–150
    partner receiving nude photos from other men and, 162–164
    sleeves for, 150, 157
    strokes and hand use, 149
    vibrators and (See vibrators)
        medical/doctor fetishes, 120
        missionary position, 62
        missionary position with vibrating cock ring, 176

N

negativity about sex
    lies, misinformation and, 10–11
    shame and, 9–10
NEMO (non-ejaculatory multiple orgasm), 172
"no means no," 16–17, 133
nudes. See photos, nude

BEST. SEX. EVER.

O

obesity, ED and, 80
oil-based lubes, 61, 107
oils as lubes, 153
open-legged spoon position, 90
oral sex
    best ever (testimonials), 56
    best positions for blowjobs, 54–55
    best positions for vulva, 52–53
    double oral position, 137
    eating ass, 110–113
    going down on a vulva, 50, 52–53
    small penis size and, 86
    standing O position, 91
    upping your game, 50–51
orgasms, 165–180. *See also* ejaculation
    about
        defined, 168
    blended, 175
    denying, 130
    difference between prostate and penile (confessions), 173
    hacking, 166
    inability to have (anorgasmia), 167, 179
    lasting longer and, 48, 81–83
    multiple, with penis, 169–172
    non-ejaculatory multiple (NEMO), 172
    prostate, 170–171, 173
    refractory period and, 169, 171, 172
    Sexplain It column (Needs Release), 178–180
    universal rules for making someone cum, 166–167
outercourse, 49

P

pearly gates position, 91
pegging, 67, 69, 101, 109
pelvic-floor muscles, 81–82, 148
pelvis pillow, 65
penis
    best positions for meaty ones, 90–91
    best positions for small ones, 88–89
    Big Dick Energy (BDE) cultivation, 93–94
    blood flow issues, 79–80
    jelqing, 87
    sensitivity issues (*See* performance)
    Sexplain It column (Looking for the Right Fit), 92–94
    sheaths to increase size, 86
    size of, 84–94, 159
    small, 86–89, 92–94
    squeezing, to delay ejaculation, 82
    toys buyers guide, 156–157 (*See also* specific toys)
performance
    alcohol, drugs and, 77, 80
    anxiety, causes and dealing with, 76–78
    ED medications and, 74, 78
    erectile dysfunction (ED) and, 74–75, 79–80
    feedback on (Sexplain It column), 194–196
    lasting longer, 48, 81–83
    making others cum and pressure on, 167
    medical issues and, 79–80
    relationship problems and, 77
    religious/societal sex negativity and, 77

INDEX

seeing a doctor about, 75
stress and, 76-77
whiskey dick and, 80
perineum (taint), stimulating, 51, 53, 109, 111, 148-149
photos, nude
    asking for, 38
    getting artsy with, 38-39
    starting slowly, 35
    storing, 39
    taking selfies (best positions), 39, 40-41
    unsolicited dick pic, 39
Play, Kenneth, about, 165
pole position, 88
porn
    addiction to, assessing, 151
    ethical, 161
    myths perpetuated by, 159-161
    watching with partner, 155
positions, categories of
    anal sex, not doggy style, 114-115
    blowjobs, 54-55
    bringing vulva-owners to climax, 176-177
    classics, 62-63
    cuddling, 190-191
    eating ass, 112-113
    making sex work for your body, 64-65
    oral sex on a vulva, 52-53
    people with meaty hog, 90-91
    people with small peen, 88-89
    threesomes, 136-139
    when you're tired AF, 26-27
positions, specific
    anilingus 69, 113
    baby monkey, 191
    butt to butt, 191
    butterfly, 176
    captain, 114
    classic DP (double penetration), 138
    closed for business, 53
    coital alignment technique (CAT), 176
    cowgirl, 62
    doggy blowjob, 139
    doggy deluxe, 137
    doggy style, 63, 112
    doggy train, 136
    double cowgirl, 136
    double oral, 137
    Eiffel Tower/spit roast, 138
    extended reverse cowgirl, 115
    face-off, 64
    face-sitter (blowjob), 54
    face-sitting (anal), 113
    flat iron, 26
    gift wrapped, 26
    G-whiz, 88
    half spoon, 190
    happy baby pose, 115
    heir to the throne, 52
    horizontal hug, 190
    hot seat, 64
    hump and blow, 54
    Kivin method, 53
    lap nap, 191

launchpad, 90
   legs on shoulders, 115
   locked and loaded, 26
   lying blow, 55
   missionary, 62
   missionary with vibrating cock ring, 176
   open-legged spoon, 90
   pearly gates, 91
   pole position, 88
   pretzel, 89
   put your leg in the air, 52
   reverse cowgirl, 65
   reverse face-sit, 113
   rim shot, 112
   roly-poly, 53
   sideways 69, 54
   69, 63
   69 train, 137
   socket, 27
   spider-man, 55
   spooning, 63
   spread eagle, 89
   squatting cowgirl, 115
   stand and deliver, 65
   standing date, 55
   standing O, 91
   train (daisy chain), 139
   Venus butterfly, 177
   zodiac, 114
pretzel position, 89
prostate
   about
      illustrated, 98
   anal play and, 116, 118
   cancer, reducing risk of, 152
   masturbation and, 170–171
   orgasms, 170–171, 173
   prostate orgasms vs. penile orgasms (confessions), 173
   stimulating, 107, 170–171
   toys to reach P-spot, 108–109, 170–171
prostate massagers, 67, 69, 109, 156
P-spot, 98, 170–171
pubococcygeal (PC) muscles, strengthening, 81–82, 169. *See also* edging
put your leg in the air position, 52

R

reasons we have sex, 6–7
reverse cowgirl position, 65
reverse face-sit position, 113
rim shot position, 112
role play, 129
roly-poly position, 53

S

sadomasochism, 121–122. *See also* BDSM
safe word, 125, 133
self-love. *See* masturbation
sex. *See also* specific topics
   positions (*See* positions, categories of; positions, specific)
   prepping bed for, 184
   reasons we have, 6–7

INDEX

tips for after (*See* after sex)
weight of shame and, 9–10
sex party tips for newbies, 140–142. *See also* threesomes and group sex
sex toys. *See also* butt plugs; cock rings; dildos; prostate massagers; vibrators
   about
      overview of, 66–67
   anal toys, 108–109
   buyers guides, 68–69, 108–109, 156–157
   cleaning after sex, 185
   clitoris and, 66–67, 69, 94, 150
   gender-affirming, finding, 67
   outercourse and, 49
   partner preferring toy to you, 66–67
   penis toys, 156–157
   to use as a couple, 68–69
   ways to use, 67
Sexplain It columns
   about, 11
   Bad Student, 194–196
   Failed Dirty Talker, 45–46
   Just Wants Head, 70–72
   Kinky in Florida, 143–144
   Looking for the Right Fit, 92–94
   Needs Release, 178–180
   Obsessed With Anal, 116–118
   Old and Boring, 28–30
   Trouble in Paradise, 162–164
sexting
   confessions, 37
   nudes (taking, sending, storing) and, 38–41
   prompts to use, 35–36
   starting dirty talk with, 34–35
   unsolicited dick pic, 39
   writing sexy story, 36
sexually transmitted infections (STIs), avoiding, 57–59, 159–160
sheaths, penis, 86
sideways 69 position, 54
silicone-based lubes, 61, 99, 107
Sinclair, Alicia, about, 95
69 position, 63. *See also* anilingus 69 position; sideways 69 position
69 train position, 137
sleep, masturbation and, 152–153
sleeves, masturbation, 150, 157
socket position, 27
spider-man position, 55
spit vs. lube, 61, 99
spooning position, 63. *See also* half spoon position; open-legged spoon position
spread eagle position, 89
squatting cowgirl position, 115
squirting, 160, 177
stand and deliver position, 65
standing date position, 55
standing O position, 91
stress
   cuddling reducing, 189
   masturbation releasing, 152
   performance and, 76–77
submissive roles, 54, 97, 109, 120, 123, 127, 129
switches (both dominant and submissive), 127

T

taint. *See* perineum
Taylor, Jordyn, about, 11
testosterone, low, ED and, 80
threesomes and group sex, 132–139
    about
        overview of, 132
    best ever (testimonials), 135
    checking with participants after, 134
    discussing, 133
    most awkward experience (confessions), 142
    "no" and, 133
    positions you can totally pull off, 136–139
    preparing for, 133
    rules and boundaries, 133
    safe word for, 133
    setting boundaries, 133, 140–142
    sex party tips for newbies, 140–142
    unicorns and, 139
    what to do during, 134
timing of sex, mismatched desires, 24–25
toys. *See* sex toys
train position (daisy chain), 139

U

unicorns, 139

V

vampire kiss, 21
variety, importance of, 7
Venus butterfly position, 177
vibrating cock rings, 67, 157, 176
vibrators, 62, 66–67, 69, 149, 150, 157, 176
voyeurism, 124
vulva. *See also* clitoris
    bringing vulva-owners to climax, 176–177
    going down on, 50
    outercourse and, 49
    reaching orgasm with, 174–175
    squirting and, 160, 177

W

water-based lubes, 61, 99
whiskey dick, 80
why we have sex, 6–7

Z

Zane, Zachary, about, 11
zodiac position, 114

BEST. SEX. EVER.

**HEARST
HOME**

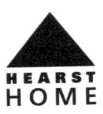

Copyright © 2022 by Hearst Magazines, Inc.

All rights reserved. The written instructions in this volume are intended for the personal use of the reader and may be reproduced for that purpose only. Any other use, especially commercial use, is forbidden under law without the written permission of the copyright holder.

This book is intended as a reference volume only, not a medical manual. The information given here is designed to help you make informed decisions about your health. It is not intended as a substitute for any treatment that may have been prescribed by your doctor. If you suspect that you have a medical problem, we urge you to seek competent medical help.

Cover and book design by Might Could
Illustrations on pages 39, 61, 68-69, 98, 108-109, 156-157 by Might Could
All other illustrations by Alexandra Folino

Library of Congress Cataloging-in-Publication Data Available on request

10 9 8 7 6 5 4 3 2 1

Published by Hearst Home, an imprint of Hearst Books/
Hearst Communications, Inc.
300 W 57th Street
New York, NY 10019

Men's Health is a registered trademark of Hearst Magazines, Inc. Hearst Home, the Hearst Home logo, and Hearst Books are registered trademarks of Hearst Communications, Inc.

For information about custom editions, special sales, premium and corporate purchases:
hearst.com/magazines/hearst-books

Printed in The United States of America
ISBN 978-1-950785-87-2